Yes, Real Women Do Sweat;
Straight Talk About Menopause

By

Linda Hawkins

Published by

DoriNu Publications, LLC
Dayton, OH
DorindaDENusum.com

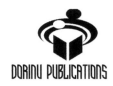

DORINU PUBLICATIONS

Published by DoriNu Publications, LLC

DoriNu Publications, LLC
Dayton, OH
DorindaDENusum.com

ISBN-13: 978-0-9835662-4-3
ISBN-10: 0983566240

Cover by Charlotte Brown
Edited by Dorinda D. E. Nusum

Printed in the United States of America

ACKNOWLEDGEMENTS

First and foremost, I want to thank God for the vision of developing this guidebook. I realize that these unique ideas came as a result of Him and not from me. Secondly, I want to acknowledge my husband, Sylvester who encouraged me to try my hand at writing. He knew how important it was to me to share with women what I know about health and wellness and he suggested putting my information in a book. He even purchased an e-book for me to study which provided modules with valuable techniques on how to create a professional book. Thank you from the bottom of my heart and I love you very much.

Last, but not least, I want to thank a friend who is really dear to me. She has mentored, coached and encouraged me every step of the way and that is LaTonya Branham who is also an accomplished author. Thank you for being there for me "Tonya" and always believing in me. Your words of encouragement and slight push, kept me going when it was really easy to give up. You are the best. Much success to you.

CHAPTER 1

WHY THIS BOOK CAME ABOUT

When I woke up this morning I asked myself, "What is life about?" I found the answer in my room...the fan said, "Be cool." The roof said, "Aim high." The window said, "See the world!" The clock said, "Every minute is precious." The mirror said, "Reflect before you act." The calendar said, "Be up to date." The door said, "Push hard for your goals." The floor said, "Kneel down and pray. - Author unknown

This book came about as a result of women who approached me while at their wits end with what to do regarding this thing called menopause. I kept hearing common questions, such as, "How can I begin to feel normal again and why am I sad or angry the majority of the time? What do I do when the hot flashes hit and how do I avoid them? What does it mean when I have irregular periods? Why do I sweat every night? Why can't I sleep at night and why am I so tired every day?" Last but not least, "Am I going crazy because everything leads to that direction" These are just a few of the common questions that women over 40 are asking. If you are not asking yet, just keep living because very few women are immune.

Subsequently, I was compelled to create a handbook that would answer many of their questions. By addressing these questions I will assist women with understanding their journey and how to travel through it in a positive manner. It is still possible to live a quality life. It is time for some straight talk.

While addressing some of the questions I have encountered over the years, my ultimate goal is to empower women. Women need to believe that being 40+ does not mean they are coming to the end of their lives. On the contrary, it's just beginning. Several people talk about this being the "second chance" life, or part two of their existence. It is time to enjoy and experience part two to its fullest. Today you have shed baggage from those early years. Look at it this way, you no longer have to deal with those worrisome menstrual periods.

I was in the pharmacy a few weeks ago and noticed the hygiene products and realized that I do not have to spend money buying those sanitary products anymore. I don't have to concern myself with what time of the month it is, whether I should wear white clothes, you know the rest. Those days are over. How empowering that feels.

Most of us are empty nesters, near retirement or ready to embark upon the next adventure. Wherever you are in your journey it can be liberating. It is time to demonstrate your "second chance" power. Travel, write a book (like I did) be creative, join a cause, start your own business. The possibilities are limitless.

Remember, if you don't do it now then when? You don't get a third chance. So you see this book is so much more than facts about Menopause.

If you are a Baby Boomer this book is dedicated to you. Currently Baby Boomers are one of the most valued segments -of the population. Statistics tell us that there are over 76 million Baby Boomers - individuals born between1946 and 1964 reaching between 48 and 66 years old, "[1] This means many Baby Boomers are moving towards menopause, experiencing its fullest state or moving into the post menopausal stage. Either way, they are all menopausal and a force to reckon with. As the Baby-Booming population ages, it is estimated that more than 5,000 American women each day reach menopause.[2] The statistics are staggering, thus, my urgency in writing this book.

In my opinion every female and male over 30 years old should have this book in his or her hands. In addition, this book serves to let the world know that it is womanly or ladylike to sweat. Women have earned the right to sweat whether they are pumping iron, running a race or sitting and reading a book. There is no shame in it because it is a natural occurrence. It is as natural as having hunger pangs when your brain sends messages to your stomach that you are hungry. So, ladies, when you begin to sweat you no longer have to be ashamed because *Yes, Real Women do Sweat.*

It is my hope this book will elicit open dialogue between women. There is a section in the book that focuses on how this topic is taboo. It is seen as taboo because most women are fearful to openly discuss it. Not only should we discuss it with our friends and family we should talk with our doctors about it. Ask them questions and don't stop until you get good answers that you are totally satisfied with. As long as it remains taboo, women will remain ignorant about this phase of their lives, they will continue to suffer needlessly and they will have very little power. Remember, this guide is about empowering women.

Last, but certainly not least of all, I wanted to provide a gift to the men who will endure some bumps and bruises during the menopausal stages. Understand that you are on this journey also. You will encounter several different women in one (split personality) as your mate goes through her journey. You will freeze, get snapped at, feel unloved, lose a lover, be a moving target sometimes all in the same day, but you must hang in there. It's imperative to remain strong and supportive.

Men, read this book, take notes, highlight important

points, use it as your guide through menopause. But don't stop there. Read other materials so you can gain a total understanding of what your love one is going through. Believe me by doing this it will strengthen your love and your relationship. Just remember it really is not about you. It's all about; "REAL WOMEN DO SWEAT" and so will your mate.

It has been a real pleasure writing on this topic. I wanted to deal with it plainly and I hope I've accomplished what I set out to do. I don't have all the answers, but neither do the medical experts who are still trying to figure out perimenopause, menopause and post menopause. Unfortunately, there is so little money being put into research of understanding this vital phase of a women's life. But, as new things are discovered more and more women will experience relief.

"This is a new generation of midlife women. You have never seen so many beautiful women over 50 in your lifetime. This generation has it all; beauty, brains and wisdom."- Linda Hawkins

ABOUT THE "HER STORIES"

Throughout the book I have provided real, authentic, stories that you'll find genuinely relevant, as their story may be similar to or identical to your story. Be reassured that these women are bona fide, with real hot flashes, real mood swings and real sweat to share and talk about. Their names have been changed to protect the innocent.

My rationale for having them share their story is to encourage you, while giving you hope to move forward and to continue putting one foot in front of the other. But more importantly, to confirm that you are not alone in this journey others have gone through some incredible occurrences and are still standing. It may also confirm that yes there is something wrong with you, but it's normal. It will also confirm that no matter what society tries to imply, that real women truly do sweat. The interviewees range from perimenopause to postmenopausal, ranging from 48-80+years old. It is my belief that this component of the book enhances the information that I am offering in each chapter. In some cases it is not necessary for me to elaborate or even address particular topics for the reason that the "Her stories" may cover it sufficiently.

I do not expect for you to receive from these interviews medical facts. On the contrary, for each woman, the facts are experiential. So, understand these are not considered as factual in nature, but they are valuable in nature because it is truth - her truth. It was my intent to leave the wording as raw and original as possible, but in a few cases, it was necessary for me to reword or rephrase for readability. What a wealth of experiences, knowledge and wisdom was gained through the writings! It is my hope that you enjoy reading the womens' stories as much as I enjoyed my time with them while capturing and sharing their experiences.

"A sure way for one to lift himself up is by helping to lift someone else." - Booker T. Washington

CHAPTER 2

DEFINING MENOPAUSE 101

"Educate a man and you educate an individual…educate a woman and you educate a nation. - African Proverb

There will come a time in a woman's life when she will experience physical, mental and emotional upheaval. This change begins in her mid to late 40's while she is busy raising children, climbing the corporate ladder, volunteering in the community, and so on. To this end she may not be totally conscious of those subtle changes that are occurring in her body. Fundamentally, the changes are not drastic but they do exist all because of a lower level of hormones being manufactured by the body such as estrogen and progesterone. As she matures, those subtleties become more pronounced. More than anything, this is a sign that she is shifting from one season into another, from spring to fall and for some from fall to winter.

Why do we change? It is quite simple. When a woman no longer has a menstrual period for at least 12 months and she does so without any interruption, she is officially in the menopausal stage. "Menopause actually means the end of menstruation….you aren't officially menopausal until you haven't had a period for a year."[3]

Without a doubt if you are 50 years old or older, you are either in or getting ready to enter into one of the menopausal phases. This includes mothers, grandmothers, sisters and aunts, all races, nationalities or color. There is no discrimination. All Women will cease manufacturing their estrogen and progesterone hormones.

It also affects young women such as, 20 through 40-year olds who had to have "female" surgery. There will be more discussion on premature menopause later in this book.

Menopause manifests itself at different times in each woman's life. Many women do not understand what is transpiring when perimenopause or even menopause begins, so they are unable to pinpoint its beginnings.

Furthermore, they experience the symptoms but, can't interpret them because they have not been taught the beginning or advanced characteristics of menopause.

Unfortunately, if they were asked when this event began, they wouldn't be able to pinpoint it. Many can recall when and where their first hot flash experience took place, or irregularity of their menstrual period, but that is probably the extent of their recollection.

My non-clinical description of perimenopause or menopause is; sometimes looks like a vicious, ugly hairy animal with fangs and claws and very dangerous. It can be impatient and curt with loved ones. Sometimes, it is sultry, wimpy, mushy, thinned skinned, while just trying to make it through the day without crying her eyes out. At times she is in a fog, perplexed, confused and having difficulty making heads or tails of it all with her inability recollecting anything that she knew last year, or even last week. Despite witnessing numerous personalities that look differently at any given time, it's still your mother, wife, sister, or friend just trying to make sense out of what is happening to her and how to remain normal through it all. Menopause exists within the mind, body and spirit. Essentially the mind, because of the mental aspects involved.

For example, women experience depression, sadness, moodiness, fogginess, and many other emotions, which temporarily affect their mental wellbeing. They try to wrap their brains around what is happening. This is equally so with the body, as there are a number of physical changes that one experiences, which sometimes is discerning, like the inconsistency and duration of a woman's menstrual flow, stiff or sore joints, headaches, shifting body weight, and slow metabolism, hence making it difficult to lose those extra pounds, or dislike her body. I could go on.

Similarly, spiritual demeanor is tested, through mood swings, depression or sadness. There's unhappiness with self and likewise with others around women. They develop a lack of a sense of interconnectedness with all living creatures; lack of awareness of the purpose and meaning of life, and no inner peace in life.[4] In cases such as those, *"Self help is the best help"- AESOP-from Hercules and Wagoner*

Most women do not prepare for Menopause so it comes as a big surprise. It sneaks up gradually. Sometimes this happens without their even knowing what happened. The symptoms are there, but not in the forefront of their lives, not yet anyway. Because they were not in tune to their bodies, the symptoms hit women like a ton of bricks.

For some women, menopausal symptoms come fast and furious and they are miserable, stressed and depressed. They basically go into a deep funk and need major intervention to get out of it. For others, it could come quietly and unassumingly. Why does it happen? That is a million dollar question that only can be answered by the divine one. It happens because that is how God destined women to travel through the aging process.

A woman's body is architected like a well designed machine (actually better than a machine). For many years, it provides housing to fertilize an egg, procreate up until approximately 48 yrs of age and then the ovulation slowly, but methodically comes to a complete stop and the body turns that baby-making machine off, so women can move on to their next stage. That stage also includes the decreasing of the hormone's estrogen and progesterone. Estrogen protects your bones and cardiovascular system among other responsibilities .[5]

How long must women go through this you ask? Well, there is very little research done about the length of the menopausal period. If you ask a woman who is going through it, her response would be, "Too long". Some experts say the perimenopausal stage is a 10 year period. However, several women who I have spoken with have been experiencing their symptoms for more than 10 years. Some have had hot flashes for over 15-20 years. It appears that it really depends on the person. There is no real timetable or start time, nor ending time. Some believe, that if women started their periods early (10-12 years old), they will stop their menstrual cycles early, but there isn't enough data to support that theory.

Mansfield et al. (2004) explain that there is considerable variation in the women's movement across menopausal status categories, so much so that researchers have to be ready to reject the notion of a regular progression from perimenopause to menopause to postmenopause or a regular menopausal age or duration and to search for a broader conceptualization of menopause in future studies. In one longitudinal study of 100 women that took place over the span of 3–12 years, some women lasted in one stage for numerous years and then moved on quickly, some flip-flopped between stages over many years, and some progressed quickly through all three clinically defined stages.

Definitions of the 4 Menopausal Stages

1. Premature Menopause

Because nature is designed to operate on its own timetable when something occurs before its time, it's defined as premature. Our bodies have a biological clock designed to time when we'll begin going through the change of life, unless, of course, it happens earlier, such as, in our 20's or 30's, which is considered premature. Items that can cause premature changes are: surgery, illnesses, and obesity, just to name a few. Surgical removal of both ovaries, also called a bilateral oophorectomy (OH-uh-fuh-REK-tuh-mee), causes menopause right away. A woman's periods will stop after this surgery, and her hormones drop quickly. She may immediately have strong menopausal symptoms such as hot flashes and diminished sexual desire.

Some women who have a hysterectomy (his-tur-EK-tuh-mee), which removes the uterus, are able to keep their ovaries. They will not enter menopause right away because their ovaries will continue to make hormones. But, because their uterus is removed, they no longer have their periods and cannot get pregnant. They might have hot flashes because the surgery can sometimes affect the blood supply to the ovaries. Later on, they might have natural menopause a year or two earlier than expected. [6] Radical Hysterectomy removes the uterus, cervix, ovaries, fallopian tubes, and possibly upper portions of the vagina. Apparently, many women are choosing this procedure because of cancer, or trouble with their ovaries, and their doctors may determine it best for removal. The United States has the highest rate of hysterectomies in the industrialized world, and according to the Centers for Disease Control and Prevention (CDC), hysterectomy is the second most frequently performed surgical procedure (after cesarean sections) for U.S. women. Approximately 600,000   hysterectomies are performed annually in the United States, and approximately 20 million American women have had a hysterectomy.[7]

2. Perimenopause

Perimenopause occurs when the body is naturally set in motion to change, usually between the ages of 40-48. During that time, women will begin experiencing some midlife changes, such as, hot flashes, memory lapses, mood swings, uneasiness and so on. Better put, "Perimenopause refers to the time leading up to the cessation of menstruation, when estrogen production is slowing down. A lot of the symptoms that folks usually label as "menopausal" actually take place during the perimenopausal years." A woman's period is late at this time, because her ovaries produce less estrogen during the first part of her normal cycle or because she may never have ovulated, making the entire cycle weird and unusual, sometimes heavy, sometimes light."[9]

3. Menopause

Menopause happens when the menstrual cycle has ceased and women experience several symptoms. Their bodies are now beginning to go through a process, a journey that ends only after there has been no menstrual period for 12 consecutive months. Yet, there is no set fast rule. As a woman's body is ever changing, even after 12 months, she could experience a menstrual period or spotting, so it is recommended that one additional year should be added to be considered full menopause. It should be noted that Dr. Northrup, international author on women's health, warns that it is possible to get pregnant during both of these phases.[10]

4. Post Menopause

Technically, the time after menopause is called postmenopausal, but this word has never really caught on. So, in keeping with common usage, we most often use the term menopause to refer to the actual event and the years after menopause. We use post menopause only when it helps to clarify things. Once a woman has reached menopause, she enters into a postmenopausal state. Postmenopause refers to all the years after menopause or more simply stated, all the remaining years of a woman's life. During this stage, hormone levels can continue to decline. Therefore, symptoms caused by a reduction of hormone levels may continue for a few years until some symptoms no longer exist. According to the North American Menopause Society, an American woman spends one-third to one-half of her life in postmenopause.[11]

"Life is like an enormous room in which somebody keeps moving the furniture; you can't tell from moment to moment whether you're about to plop into your favorite easy chair or a potted cactus."-Eric V. Copage

15

Her Story 1 – Dana

I remarried in 1969 with 3 children in tow. Four years later, my daughter died in a fatal car crash, and then in 1979 I lost my father. Things were going well until 2000 when I lost 2 grandchildren. Shortly after those incidents, I started to take care of my mother, approximately from 2002 until 2007, when she was diagnosed with breast cancer. She passed away that same year.

It seemed as if I was always taking care of someone else and never had time for me. The year of her passing I was diagnosed with breast cancer and began chemotherapy. Then, in 2009, because I had so much pain in my chest, neck, and shoulders, I went into the hospital for pleurisy, but while in there the doctors discovered a reoccurrence of the breast cancer. Now, in 2011, I am once again receiving chemo treatments, although I don't know how long I have to take them.

Of course, all of this is a lot to contend with, but one year, my friend paid for me to attend a Christian retreat in Tennessee, which increased my faith in man and in God.

I grew up in the church and learned about God, but being on a mountain with just women who were teachers of God's word made me understand better how God really works. If it hadn't been for that I don't think I could have survived everything that I went through. I learned that everything He does is for my good because God doesn't make mistakes. He placed me in one level while preparing me for another level. I learned in order to make it through my trials and tribulations, I had to lean on Him.

I was in my late 40s when I discovered I was experiencing menopause. My first symptom was experiencing warmth in my feet. The warmth started in my feet and traveled up my legs to my knees and then all the way up my upper body. It was as if a heated blanket had been placed over me and it caused me to sweat, which was unusual for me. This no longer happens. Now, I just get a little sweaty on the top of my head.

Secondly, I was very moody. Everything would get on my nerves. I was especially moody while I was having a hot flash, but after the hot flash my moodiness would go away. I didn't really *have night sweats, just day sweats. During the stage of my sweating, I became aware of how sugar causes hot flashes. One of my church members brought it to my attention. I was eating a peppermint and she said that the peppermint would cause me to experience a hot flash. At the time, I did not believe there was a connection, so I decided to test her theory a couple days later. After eating a small peppermint, I had a hot flash just as she said I would.*

As I mentioned earlier, my feet would get very hot and I went to the doctor and told him I was having hot flashes and I need something for it. I had to work and I couldn't let this interfere. I don't think he took me very seriously because he responded, "Well I don't know what I can give you for it". I told him if he didn't give me anything, headlines would read: Lady Kills Doctor Over Hot Flashes, so he found something to prescribe.

The first prescription was a temporary fix. It helped for a short while, but the symptoms returned. Then, he put me on Premarin, for 10 years and then Provera. I took two different pills for years and later, my doctor discovered Primpro, which I took instead of the other two medications. I took 1 pill for 3 years and I can't say I have a bad experience, compared to other people.

I want to know when this is going to stop. I have learned to adjust. When I'm rushing around and hot flashes come, I have to slow down. My recommendation to other women is to ask questions. I failed to ask the right questions. Women should also read books to gain knowledge to understand their bodies. Now, there are more books about menopause. When I was growing up, discussing menopause was taboo. We just didn't talk about it.

"There does not have to be powerlessness. The power is within ourselves"-Faye Wattleton

---

CHAPTER 3

MENOPAUSE SYMPTOMS-MORE THAN HOTFLASHES

There are several commonalities to menopause and they are the many symptoms that each and every woman will experience. Women will not experience all of them, but they could feasibly experience more than one simultaneously. For example, she could experience hot flashes and heart palpitations at the same time or mood swings and anxiety attacks together. Symptoms are like Rights of Passage for women. In comparison, when girls or teens first began their menstrual cycle they were defined by some as women. In fact, in some countries, they would be offered to their prospective husband because they would be considered ready to marry and bear children.

Below is a non all-inclusive list of symptoms with brief definitions. If you are not experiencing any of these items listed, I believe it is safe to say you are not menopausal.

- Hot Flashes - When the body heats up to an uncomfortable temperature and may induce sweating
- Dry and Thin Vaginal Walls - Walls of the vaginal area are extremely dry causing occasional itching, pain and discomfort during intercourse
- Anxiety - Physical and or emotional experiences of fear, and shallow breathing, attacks that are uncontrollable

- Mood Swings - To go from a good mood to a very bad mood in a short period of time with no forewarning
- Heart Palpitations - When the heart physically pumps faster than usual. Can happen without warning and for little to no reason at all
- More susceptible to various cancers
- High Risk ofHeart Disease - Number one killer of women over 50
- Osteoporosis - as a result of low calcium and vitamin D in the body, this bone disease is present
- Depression - emotionally being in a deep dark place
- Low Libido - sex drive is little to none
- Arthritis and Sore Joints - Joints tend to be stiff and sore
- Dry or Itchy skin – must use creams or lotions to find comfort
- Night Sweats - similar to hot flashes, but sweat more profusely while sleeping
- Insomnia - experience restless to no sleeping and waking up often with an inability to get back to sleep
- Foggy Thinking or Forgetfulness - All of a sudden you cannot remember the simplest things or you find yourself losing your train of thought
- Dry Eyes - eyes tend to be dry and itchy often
- Facial Hair - signs of hair popping out under and around your chin
- Craving of Sugar and Carbohydrates - You crave these items more than usually
- Urinary Tract Infections - without warning you have that embarrassing leak
- Weight Gain - middle-aged weight which is difficult to shed. It has been said that women gain an average of 10 pounds per year.

Next, in this section, the objective is to explain each symptom listed above. The more familiar women become with them, the more likely they will be to determine normalcy, opposed to whether or not she needs to seek medical attention.

Some of our issues can rightfully be filed under **M** for menopause, while other symptoms may have to be looked after by a physician. The purpose of this book is to help women to determine the difference, but when in doubt…seek professional help.

Decisions must be made to address hormonal imbalances to achieve complete health and wellness and to decide whether to seek hormonal therapy or use holistic methods. Some of the alternatives are; healthy eating, taking herbs and vitamins or exercising. The key is to do something. There is no reason for a woman to suffer through this period of her life or to cause her family to suffer.

"Don't worry about failure-think about the chances you miss when you don't even try!"- Anonymous

❖ **Hot flashes** – It is usually the first thing people think of when menopause is mentioned, mainly because it is one symptom that is physically visible to you and other people. If you've had one, there's no mistaking it- 'the sudden, intense, hot feeling on your face and upper body, perhaps preceded or accompanied by a rapid heartbeat and sweating, nausea, dizziness, anxiety, headache, weakness, or a feeling of suffocation. Some women report that they knew they were about to have the experience before it happened. An aura, or premonition, may feel like nausea, or a tingling or pressing sensation in the head. Some women become weak in the knees or dizzy and have to sit down. The upper body from the chest to the scalp, may begin to sweat profusely.[11]

The flash is followed by a flush, leaving women reddened and perspiring. That is why some refer to it as a hot flush. Women can have a soaker or merely a moist upper lip. A chill can lead off the episode or be the finale.

A diminished level of estrogen has a direct effect on the hypothalamus, the part of the brain responsible for controlling your appetite, sleep cycles, sex hormones, and body temperature. Somehow, (we don't know how), the drop in estrogen confuses the hypothalamus — which is sometimes referred to as the body's "thermostat" — and makes it read "too hot."

The brain responds to this report by broadcasting an all-out alert to the heart, blood vessels, and nervous system: "Get rid of the heat!" The message is transmitted by the nervous system's chemical messenger. The message is delivered instantly. Women's hearts pumps faster, the blood vessels in their skin dilate to circulate more blood to radiate off the heat, and their sweat glands release sweat to cool them off even more. Some women's skin temperature can rise six degrees centigrade during a hot flash. Their bodies cool down when it shouldn't, and they are miserable: soaking wet in the middle of a board meeting or in the middle of a good night's sleep.[12]

❖ **Dry and thin vaginal walls** - As a result of a low level of estrogen, the vaginal area tends to be dry, scratchy, may itch excessively and at sometimes can be painful. Estrogen, a female hormone, helps keep vaginal tissue healthy by maintaining a normal vaginal acidity level. Acidity creates a natural defense against vaginal and urinary tract infections. But when your estrogen levels decrease, so does this natural defense and the amount of vaginal lubrication. According to Drs. M. P. Brincat & J. Calleja-Agius, "With estrogen loss, the vagina shortens and narrows due to the loss of elasticity and ruguae, and thinning of its walls." Dyspareunia and vaginal bleeding from fragile atrophic skin are common problems. [13] When the vaginal mucosa is well estrogenized, it is called "cornified epithelium". Cornified refers to cells that are tough and resilient. After menopause, some women lose the outer cornified layers of their vaginal tissue.[14] The point is, many women suffer from an extremely dry and irritated vaginal area. Left untreated, vaginal atrophy can result in years of vulvovaginal discomfort, with a significant impact on quality of life.[15]

Those who are sexually active may experience great discomfort and sometimes painful irritation. Regular washing with a moisturizing cream is often the most helpful for vulval irritation and dryness. Women experiencing recurrent urinary tract infections should be instructed that consumption of pure cranberry lingon berry juice will decrease their risk of urinary tract infections [16]

Three valuable recommendations from The North American Menopause Society to deal with vaginal atrophy include:

1. The primary goals of vaginal atrophy management are to relieve symptoms and reverse atrophic anatomic changes
2. First line therapies for women with vaginal atrophy include non-hormonal vaginal lubricants and moisturizers.
3. For symptomatic vaginal atrophy that does not respond to nonhormonal vaginal lubricants and moisturizers prescription therapy may be required.[17] For example Estrace(estradiol) is a bioidentical estrogen cream that works well for treatment of vaginal dryness, thinning and other symptoms[18]

❖   **Anxiety -** Characteristics of anxiety can be described as: comes on suddenly, hard to control, desire to lash out at others, feeling of discomfort with self, and nervousness or easily aggravated. While the English Dictionary defines it as: *"feeling of worry, nervousness or agitation, often about something that is going to happen. Something that worries* *somebody."* Anxiety may come upon people without any warning and they might find themselves showing aggression towards friends and family with no apparent cause. Women may also experience anxiety along with hot flashes, night sweats and depression. These symptoms seem to work hand in hand. The first step is to recognize she is having an anxiety attack. Once she recognizes it, she should use techniques to calm herself down. There are several stress relievers or stress management techniques available.

❖ **Mood Swings** - Next to hot flashes and depression this is probably the most difficult symptom to endure. No, women, you are not going crazy but you may feel as if you are. The first step is to understand mood swings and then deal with them. The same way estrogen affected you during your menstrual cycle in the form of post menstrual syndrome (PMS) is comparable because of hormone imbalance. You might fly off the handle when the smallest thing gets on your nerves or cry for every little thing?

Some women say they don't see a major difference in their moods, but those who do are convinced that they are going out of their minds and that there must be something wrong with them because of how they react from one minute to the next. The important thing to remember, women, is you are not going out of your mind. Remember it is not a mental dilemma, it's a biological issue.

Because Mood swings are a little more complex, it makes women more complex. Women should therefore, seek help and find an expert who understands the affects of low estrogen. In the meantime, they can be proactive and keep an eye on anything that may be causing mood swings, such as foods they eat, hot flashes, a stressful job, a stressful household, or life in general.

By using proactive measures and identifying the cause(s) women can begin to find ways to combat the mood changes before they come on strong. Remember, not only do these mood swings affect women, but they also affect others around them, particularly loved ones who are closest to them.

A fairly new recognized condition is perimenopause rage. This is a level above mood swings. Dr. Oz has labeled it a medical condition. It is when women for very little reason go into an uncontrollable rage and lash out at family and friends, mainly family members. Most women are apologetic after the outburst, but admit that they have no control over them.

❖ **Heart Palpitations** - Heart palpitations are accompanied by the sensation of the heart skipping a beat or beating too many times within a specific time period. Heart palpitations usually occur sporadically over a period of two to three months. Heart palpitations may accompany hot flashes, a common symptom of menopause, increasing the heart rate between 8 and 16 beats a minute. Some women have been known to experience heart rates of up to 200 beats per minute when experiencing heart palpitations. [20]

According to Dr. Marco DiBuono, of Ontario's Heart and Stroke Foundation, everyone has his or her own normal heart beat rhythm. Some are faster or slower than others. Usually, the heart beats between 60 and 80 times per minute. When people feel heart palpitations, also known as abnormal heart rhythms or arrhythmias, it is an abnormal heart rhythm for individuals. An arrhythmia may cause the heart to beat too slowly (bradycardia, less than 60 beats per minute) or too quickly (tachycardia, more than 100 beats per minute), or cause uncoordinated contractions (fibrillation). While it is important to speak to your doctor if you feel an abnormal heart rhythm, not all heart rhythm abnormalities are necessarily fatal. [20]

❖ **High risk of Heart Disease** - Coronary heart disease, often simply called heart disease, is the main form of heart disease. It is a disorder of the blood vessels of the heart that can lead to heart attack. A heart attack happens when an artery becomes blocked, preventing oxygen and nutrients from getting to the heart. [22] We should all be concerned because heart disease has become the number one deadly disease for females over the age of 55.

All of our lives estrogen has been a protector of our heart. If you are wondering why there is a high risk for middle aged women, it really is obvious. Since women no longer produce estrogen, the heart is defenseless to a negative lifestyle such as, eating unhealthy, fatty foods that clog the arteries or neglecting to exercise regularly to strengthen the heart or being overweight or obese. There are many risk factors that we know but do nothing about. All risk factors should be taken seriously and women who are over 50 should consider changing their lifestyles. Making a lifestyle change is the key to living longer, healthier lives.

The jury is still out on how to determine when a woman is having a heart attack. More research is needed. Women should learn the heart attack warning signs. These are:

1. Pain or discomfort in the center of the chest.
2. Pain or discomfort in other areas of the upper body, including the arms, back, neck, jaw, or stomach.
3. Other symptoms, such as shortness of breath, breaking out in a cold sweat, nausea, or light-headedness.

As with men, women's most common heart attack symptom is chest pain or discomfort. But women are somewhat more likely than men to experience some of the other common symptoms, particularly shortness of breath, nausea/vomiting, and back or jaw pain.[23]

These symptoms are more subtle than the obvious crushing chest pain often associated with heart attacks. This may be because women tend to have blockages not only in their main arteries, but also in the smaller arteries that supply blood to the heart — a condition called small vessel heart disease or microvascular disease" [24]

I had a very good friend die in her sleep after having a full and active day with her church friends one Saturday. Her husband said she complained of being extremely exhausted and wanted to rest a while on the couch before going to bed. She never woke up. She had a heart attack while she slept.

Her Story 2 – Jean A.

I began my Menopause experience at 45. I started so young because of female issues and was required to have surgery. My doctor warned me that I would experience menopause prematurely and recommended that I wear an estrogen patch, which I did for 6 months. But, after the 6 months, I decided to go cold turkey and do without the patch. My first symptom was not being able to sleep at night because of night sweats. I would keep a glass of ice water by my bed to drink but that resulted in having to get up often and go to the bathroom, sometimes 2-3 times a night and of course that broke my sleep. Then, I began to have hot flashes during the day, which could last 1-2 minutes. As a result I'd wear clothing that I would be able to get out of quickly. In fact, to this day, I only wear sleeveless outfits with jackets so I could disrobe swiftly if I get too hot. I noticed if I'm in a cool environment, I don't have as many hot flashes. Also, when I go into a public environment where the temperature is not comfortable, I start fanning to cool off, which I hate, but I do what I have to do. My issue is sweating. Sometimes, if women sweat too hard their clothes get sticky or makeup runs and it can be embarrassing and we feel the need to be apologetic. The problem is people in general feel women are not supposed to sweat. Even though menopause is a natural thing, most people don't see it as natural.

Most nights I sweat so badly I have stopped wearing pajamas to bed. If I do wear them, they end up off my body by the middle of the night.

Lastly, I noticed more weight gain. I believe I am one and a half sizes larger then I was before I began menopause. I was planning to lose weight for a high school reunion that was coming up, but that didn't happen. I went shopping for a new dress. I tried on a pretty red dress and took it off because when I looked in the mirror, I decided I looked like a big red tomato. So, I wore an old outfit to the reunion.

I have been going through menopause for 3 years now, two and a half of those years were without the patch. I may have 6 more years to go! Lord, have mercy. I am disappointed that it is still going on because when talking to people, some say I still have about a year to go, while others say I have about 5 yrs. Some say 8-10 years and I say, "Oh, my God, I don't know if I can make it."

My husband is the one who is most affected by the symptoms I endure. I toss and turn at night so he can't sleep either. I can understand his frustration; although, he has learned to handle it well. I would not be happy if someone kept moving around all night and interrupting my sleep. Plus, he can't sleep too close to me because he says I can't make up my mind - I want the covers on, then I throw them off. When it first started, he thought I was totally crazy, often stating, "Something is wrong with you!"

I want to maintain a healthy sex life. There are times when I felt like I could do without it. There are also times when I'm "in the mood," but fear the dryness factor. I miss the consistency of a healthy and active sex life, but it's something we have to deal with together. One thing is for sure. I should pay more attention to my body.

On occasion, vaginal dryness alters my libido, which is a strange feeling. Currently, I choose not to seek hormone replacement therapy to correct it, but I have been trying natural remedies.

Not long ago, I was watching TV and a female physician on the program said a cure for vaginal dryness is to use regular olive oil. She said, it won't hurt you when used lightly. I fear the side-effects of hormone replacement therapy (HRT), but I am willing to explore more natural remedies. I have learned to adjust to this stage of my life - no matter how crazy it seems.

❖ **Osteoporosis** - women over 50 need to be concerned with their bone density, or thickness of their bones. There are suggested numbers for bone density. Women who have low numbers stand the chance of having osteoporosis. If one has osteoporosis it means that they have fragile, brittle, bones that can break easily. Another indication is women with humps on their back. Stooped posture or kyphosis, also called a "dowager's hump". The body is robbing the calcium from the bones to support some of the others areas and so the growth appears.

The following table contains the World Health Organization's definitions of osteoporosis based on bone mineral density T-scores.

> **Normal:** Less than 1 standard deviation (SD) below the young adult reference range (more than -1)
>
> **Low bone mass (osteopoenia):** 1 to 2.5 (SDs) below the young adult reference range (-1 to 2.5)
>
> **Osteoporosis:** 2.5 or more SD's below the young adult reference range (-2.5 or less) [24]

❖ **Arthritis and sore joints** - Joints tend to be stiff and sore. Many people are experiencing this and chalking it off to old age. They believe since they are approaching 50 or 50+ that they are supposed to suffer from aching joints. But that is not necessarily true. Many things that happen to our bodies, especially our joints are self-inflicted. We do not take good care of our bodies, especially our joints. Remember, they have to carry your body around throughout your entire lifetime. These days, many people suffer from leg, knee, and hip problems and have to receive surgery to try to remove the pain and increase mobility.

Recommendation: Take Supplements such as; fish oil, Vitamin E, or Omega 3 to keep the joints lubricated. It has been recommended by the medical community that individuals over 50 should have a calcium and Vitamin D regimen for their bones, exercise 3-4 days every week unless they are trying to lose weight, then exercise more and be sure to stretch daily to decrease joint stiffness.

❖ **Depression** - Depression is a very deep dark place to be in. Today, many women suffer alone. Many don't understand what is happening to them and they are too ashamed, fearful or clueless to talk to someone about it.

Clinical depression is a serious medical illness that negatively affects how one feels, the way they think and how they act. Individuals with clinical depression are unable to function as they use to. Often, they have lost interest in activities that were once enjoyable to them, and feel sad and hopeless for extended periods of time. Clinical depression is not the same as feeling sad or depressed for a few days and then feeling better. It can affect an individual's body, mood, thoughts, and behavior. It can change their eating habits, how they feel and think, their ability to work and study, and how they interact with people. Menopausal depression can change as your hormones change. University of Health Services at Berkley explains that an examination of a 4-year cohort from this study showed that depressive symptoms increased during the menopausal transition and decreased in postmenopause[26]

If women have long periods of sadness or despair, they shouldn't delay, seek help, or talk with someone they trust. Depression not only affects you, but all of your loved ones around you. I am sure you do not want to be remembered as the mother, wife, friend or grandmother who was always depressed, or sad or difficult to be around. Women should find a friend or family member who has experienced what they are experiencing or see a professional until she gets through this period. There is nothing wrong, no matter what society says, with getting help. On the other hand, what is wrong is, suffering alone in depression without reaching out. Women must work through this stage and not just let things happen. They must be proactive fighters so they can be winners. I am a believer that food directly affects our moods.

The old adage "You are what you eat" has proven that certain foods can make you feel better, while others can have an adverse affect on you.

The items listed below contain antioxidants, designed to attack free radicals and are stress soothers;

blueberries, almonds, spinach, fresh tuna, oranges, milk, bananas, sweet potatoes, brown rice and avocado.

On the same token there are foods that have been proven to alter your mood negatively and cause you to feel anxious, bad, even sad, such as: simple carbohydrates; e.g. cakes, candy, cookies, chips refined breads, pasta. Caffeine; such as coffee, hot cocoa, teas, chocolates and of course nicotine; defined in English dictionary as (a toxic alkaloid). Each of these can affect you adversely because they contain carcinogens', caffeine and sugar.

The good news is, most people who change their diet get better within several months. Many people begin to feel better in just a few weeks.

Her Story 3 – Amber

I just realized I was suffering with menopause symptoms in the spring of 2011. My first symptom was mental imbalance. I didn't understand what was going on with me. Things were happening that were very disturbing. Sometimes I felt suicidal. Sometimes I felt lost and couldn't remember anything. I was irritable, thought I was dying. I thought I had lost my mind and needed to be committed. I often thought about being mentally evaluated by a hospital. I had gone from being a normal, happy person to totally withdrawn and messed up in the head. It was awful. I couldn't sleep. I had 3 years of total insomnia.

I stayed in a fetal position. My family doctor (who was a male) told me I was depressed. He even gave me prescriptions for depression and bipolar disorder. I cried everyday sometimes 3-4 times a day. I even went to my gynecologist (also a male) and between the two of them they drove me crazy because they kept giving me more medications, but nothing worked.

I thought of many different ways of dying. I would be driving and imagined snatching my steering wheel so I would crash into a brick wall.

I spent 3 yrs. dealing with intense hot flashes around age 49. I had heard of hot flashes, but thought it was just something that caused women to sweat. You see, I had no one to explain to me what it was like. I thought mine was a result of depression pills I was taking. Then, it kept happening at night. Even though someone suggested to me I was having hot flashes, I didn't think it could be because that was for women in their 60's or 70's. I kept thinking there had to be something wrong with me. Maybe I had a brain tumor.

Emotionally, it was the worst experience my husband has ever endured with me. He's never seen me cry and cry uncontrollably. He could not figure out what was going on and he concluded like the doctor that I was depressed. I didn't comb my hair. I didn't bathe. I didn't do anything. I would sleep all day long and stayed awake all night, as if I was afraid to sleep. It was embarrassing not being the girl he fell in love with, the woman he married or being the person he was supposed to grow old with. I had changed into someone he did not recognize. To top it off, I had to tell him that I was having suicidal thoughts, which I didn't want to tell him, but I knew if I didn't say anything I would be in big trouble.

I once thought menopause meant just the stopping of your cycle and you could no longer have children. I never thought it could do the kind of damage that could destroy marriages, families, and one's life. Things you wouldn't normally do, you would do. Before menopause, I never thought about killing myself. In   the beginning I started having vaginal irritation, so having sex was painful. My husband was sexually deprived after having a fabulous sex life with no issues. The humorous part was I was in so much pain afterwards, my vagina burned and everything hurt so I thought he had given me a sexually transmitted disease. I was thinking I was going to have to kill him because I was in so much pain.

Every time we had sex I experienced pain and I was calm about it, but in my head I was thinking that after all these years with the same man, how could I have a problem? I thought he had cheated on me and he was in big trouble. But, when I visited a new gynecologist (a female) she did several tests and reported to me that it was only menopause and that my vaginal walls were thin, dry and easy to irritate. She told me that was something she could help me to fix. Then, she prescribed the hormone therapy (HT) pills, which have changed my life.

I am glad to have my life and my mental health back. Even though I don't like medication I am just so thankful and appreciative of the HT pills because I didn't think I was going to make it through the year. I literally thought I was going to be buried. But now, I am concerned because I don't know how long I can rely on my HT to provide relief and of the side effects I will experience and what might happen to me if I get off of them. So, my fear now is this may be a temporary fix.

Since I have been going through this I have been doing research to find out more. I found out women had been institutionalized, doctors used shock treatments, and aggressive techniques used to ward out demons because men believed they were cursed all over hormonal imbalance. I think that is why *women don't talk about it. Plus, I don't think they know what's going on with them.*

I believe there should be multiple support groups in all the communities. Just like we have the organizations that focus on breast cancer, I think it is something from which all women can benefit.

❖　**Low Libido** - Although many women continue to have satisfying sex during menopause and beyond, some women experience a lagging libido during this hormonal change. There comes a time in a woman's life when intimacy is no longer a priority. For some there is little to no desire for it. Women almost forget what it feels like to love or be loved, to touch or be touched. They don't want to be caressed, embraced or even bothered. There is no such thing as foreplay, instead it is "go away".

Physical contact brings on anxiety and hot flashes and a real level of discomfort. Then, there is the issue of dry vaginal walls which can cause a double whammy — decreased interest in sex plus drier vaginal tissues, equals painful or uncomfortable sex. At the same time, women may also experience a decrease in the hormone testosterone, which boosts sex drive in men and women alike. [26]

A woman's sexual desires naturally fluctuate over the years. Highs and lows commonly coincide with the beginning or end of a relationship or with major life changes, such as pregnancy, menopause or illness. However, if you are bothered by a low sex drive or decreased sex drive, there are lifestyle changes and sex techniques that may put women in the mood more often.

So, what exactly is low sex drive in women? Experts call it Hypoactive Sexual Desire Disorder if you have a persistent or recurrent lack of interest in sex that causes you personal distress. You don't have to meet this medical definition to seek help. If you aren't as interested in sex as you'd like to be, talk to your doctor. [28]

___

Relationship issues - For many women, emotional closeness is an essential prelude to sexual intimacy. So, problems in your relationship can be a major factor in low sex drive. Decreased interest in sex is often a result of ongoing issues, such as:

- Lack of connection with your partner
- Unresolved conflicts or fights
- Poor communication of sexual needs and preference
- Infidelity or breach of trust

Symptoms of Low Libido

Obviously, the major symptom of low sex drive in women is a low or absent desire for sex. According to some studies, more than 40 percent of women complain of low sexual desire at some point.[29] Low sex drive can be very difficult for you and your partner. It's natural to feel frustrated or sad if you aren't able to be as sexy and romantic as you want — or you used to be. At the same time, low sex drive can make your partner feel rejected, which can lead to conflicts and strife. And this type of relationship turmoil can actually add to your lack of desire for sex.

It may help to remember that fluctuations in your sex drive are a normal part of every relationship and every stage of life. Try not to focus all of your attention on sex. Instead, spend some time nurturing yourself and your relationship. Go for a long walk. Get a little extra sleep. Kiss your partner goodbye before you head out the door. Make a date night at your favorite restaurant. Feeling good about yourself and your partner can actually be the best foreplay. Healthy lifestyle changes can make a big difference in your desire for sex. Here are a few helpful hints:

- **Exercise -** Regular aerobic exercise and strength training can increase your stamina, improve your body image, elevate your mood and enhance your libido.

- **Stress less** - Finding a better way to cope with work stress, financial stress and daily hassles can enhance your sex drive.

- **Be happier** - A sense of personal well-being and happiness are important to sexual interest. So find ways to bring a little extra joy to your world.

- **Strengthen your pelvic muscles** - Pelvic floor exercises (Kegel exercises) can improve your awareness of the muscles involved in pleasurable sexual sensations and increase your libido. To perform these exercises, tighten your pelvic muscles as if you're stopping a stream of urine. Hold for a count of five, relax and repeat. Do these exercises several times a day.

- **Communicate with your partner.** Conflicts and disagreements are a natural part of any relationship. Couples who learn to fight fair and communicate in an open, honest way usually maintain a stronger emotional connection, which can lead to better sex. Communicating about sex also is important. Talking about your likes and dislikes can set the stage for greater sexual intimacy.

- **Seek counseling.** Talking with a sex therapist or counselor skilled in addressing sexual concerns can help with low sex drive. Therapy often includes education about sexual response and techniques and recommendations for reading materials or couples' exercises.

- **Set aside time for intimacy.** Scheduling sex into your calendar may seem contrived and boring. But making intimacy a priority can help put your sex drive back on track.

❖ **Itchy and dry skin** - The make-up and cosmetic industry has become a multibillion dollar business helping women who are trying to preserve, regain or hang on to their youthful skin. Unfortunately, mother nature, old father time, the sun and the aging process makes it necessary to invest into facial and body creams , lotions, collagens, etc. because the skin cells are slowly dying from head to toe. Once you enter your forties, you will notice pronounced lines and wrinkles beginning to etch themselves into your skin. Collagen and elastin fibers decrease; cells retain less moisture and lose their firmness. It's time for more aggressive care [29]

To help turn dry, problem skin into smoother, supple skin, experts offer these quick tips for women in menopause:

1. **Focus on smart fats such as essential fatty acids** -- like the omega-3s found in salmon, walnuts, fortified eggs, or algae oils. These help produce your skin's oil barrier, vital in keeping skin hydrated. A diet short of these body-boosting fats can leave skin dry, itchy, and prone to acne. Most of us have a diet low in omega-3s.

2. **Smooth on sunscreen:** Keep skin healthy with "a broad spectrum sun block with an SPF of 15 or higher," says Andrea Cambio, MD, a board-certified dermatologist practicing in Cape Coral, Fla. Reflection of the sun's rays can be as intense in winter as in summer. The damage those UVA and UVB rays cause not only speeds up the skin's aging process, it can also lead to spider veins, age spots, wrinkles, and melanomas.[31]

3. **Stop those steamy showers:** Piping-hot baths and showers may feel fabulous, but hot water can be very harsh to the skin and dry it out miserably. Stop stripping your skin of its natural oils. Take shorter showers and use warm water. Also, preserve those natural oils by scrubbing with soap only in the spots you really need it, like your underarms, feet, and groin. Because your legs, back, and arms don't usually get very dirty, skip the soap and stick to a warm water wash for these areas. Take long

luxurious, warm baths with oils and moisturizes in the water. Dr. Oz, cardiovascular surgeon and talk show host, suggested we should only use soaps on those areas that naturally produce odors.

4. **Use a gentle soap:** Scented, antibacterial, or deodorant soaps can be harsh, removing your body's essential oils, leaving skin even more itchy and dry. Instead, reach for an unscented or lightly scented bar or a natural body wash with moisturizing emollients and vitamins for enrichment.

5. **Remember to moisturize:** Within a few minutes after your warm shower, smooth on your favorite moisturizer. You may favor a pricey potion from the cosmetic counter, but humbler lotions such as mineral oil and petroleum jelly help trap in much-needed moisture, also. Remember to drink lots of water. You can hydrate from the inside out by drinking water. Even though this goes without saying, it is equally important to reduce or eliminate alcohol and nicotine, both of which can prematurely age and dry the skin.

❖ **Night sweats** – These are comparable to hot flashes, but tend to produce sweat more profusely while sleeping. Night sweats is one of the most disturbing experiences you could have as a female. Some women sweat so horrific at night that they have to get up and change their soaked clothes. Others are just wet enough to wake them up out of their sleep and cause insomnia as it goes on night after night after night.

Here are four suggestions to consider that may produce some relief:

1. Be conscious of what you eat before retiring for the

night. Avoid high sugary foods, items that contain caffeine, or spicy foods. There are some fabrics that generate more heat than others such as flannel, silk, and 100% polyester or polyester blends. You may find that you sweat more when you are wearing these fabrics because they do not breathe so your body produces more heat. Select 100% cotton or a blend of 55% cotton and 45% or less of polyester. After testing this theory I can confirm its validity.

2. Also make sure the temperature of the room is cool. Your bedroom should not be cold nor do you want it hot, just a very even temperature. Years ago, my family physician recommended while sleeping, our thermostat is decreased to 65 degrees.

3. Once again, be conscious of your trigger list or know what causes hot flashes and take heed.

❖ **Insomnia** can be chronic (ongoing) or acute (short-term). Chronic insomnia means having symptoms at least 3 nights a week for more than a month. Acute insomnia lasts for less time. Some people who have insomnia may have trouble falling asleep. Other people may fall asleep easily but wake up too soon. Others may have trouble with both falling asleep and staying asleep.[31]

Some recommendations to combat insomnia are:

1. Prepare your environment for sleep - It needs to be comfortable and dark in the room. Use nightlights if afraid of the dark.
2. Follow each recommendation from the night sweats list.
3. Wind down for at least an hour prior to retiring. Listen to music or read a good book. Do something that allows you to unwind. When the

mind is racing it is hard to get to sleep and remain sleep.

4.   Get relaxed before going to bed, i.e. Take a cool relaxing bath.

5.   Reframe from eating 2-3 hours before going to bed. This allows your body time to digest your food while you are still awake. If you eat right before going to bed, your digestive system may cause insomnia or a restless night.

6.   Lastly, as mentioned earlier stay away from caffeine and sugary foods, they have stimulants that can keep you alert at the wrong time. You don't want to be alert when it is time to sleep.

❖ **Foggy thinking or forgetfulness** - All of a sudden you cannot remember the simplest things, such as remembering how to spell elementary level words or while searching for your thoughts, forgetting what you are talking about in the middle of a sentence. Sometimes forgetting procedures and steps or tasks you have been performing for years. It gets so embarrassing when you forget names of people, places and things (that you know you know). This is a devastating experience. Sometimes your thoughts are so jumbled up you have the inability to make sense of anything.

One time, while engaged in a group conversation, I was trying to say a word in order to complete a sentence, but no matter how hard I tried I could not recall this word to explain something. It was a simple and common word for me but I could not see it in my mind I could not remember it I tried to give an explanation of that word that would describe what I was trying to say but even that was a difficult task. I was so frustrated that I finally just gave up and waited for the others to change the subject.

There was another occasion when I was trying to spell a word that was familiar to me and I attempted to look it up in a paperback dictionary, but I could not get the right letters in the right order to look it up. So I decided to go online because now when using the dictionary online if you get some of the letters in the proper order it will offer you some suggestions and you can pick the word you want. Well, I could not even put enough letters in order for that to happen. Subsequently, I had to use a different word altogether. So you see, I understand what it means to be foggy. I was there once. I am so thankful that it passed.

Recommendation: No matter how frustrating the task might seem, challenge your mind. Read factual books and magazines, do crossword puzzles, research various topics and learn more about them. Involve yourself in mind games. Take classes, attend workshops. Teach what you know. Continue building those muscles in the brain so when you recover, your intellect will be sharper and smarter than ever.

This is an important chapter since it is because of forgetfulness, many women are afraid that they may be heading towards dementia or Alzheimer's. According to an expert in *Women's Body, Women's Wisdom* by Dr. Northrup, though, we must stop buying into the self-fulfilling prophecy about memory decline with age. When you are born, you have a full complement of nerve cells in your brain, which reaches its peak size at about age twenty, after which there is a gradual decline in size throughout the rest of your life. The key to appreciating and enhancing your brain function is to realize that normal loss of brain cells over time is not necessarily associated with loss of function. In fact studies have shown that throughout our lifetime, as we move from naiveté to wisdom. Our brain function becomes molded along the lines of wisdom. This is how wisdom gets wired.[33]

The great news about this menopausal symptom is it is only temporary. All of the women I have interviewed have confirmed that the forgetfulness and fogginess was only for a season. Most of them experienced what we lovingly refer to as "brain farts" for only 1-3 years. Many of them said they were in that state of mind for about 2 years. I personally experienced it for approximately 1 year. I remember so vividly when words began to come back to me. I shared with my husband that I literally felt like I had come out of a fog. I was thinking clearly once again. I am still amazed at the affects hormone imbalance has over our lives.

Her Story 4 – Cookie

I am going to be 60 this year, so I have been paying attention to the changes in my body. I really don't know exactly what is occurring but whatever they are, I believe they coincide with getting older. I don't really know what menopause is, nor do I believe I'm in it. I must admit something is going on, for example I notice a nervousness or anxiousness in me some days at work. I don't cry, but I feel like I am going to. I experience it mostly when I am overwhelmed or getting behind or someone asks me to do something. I feel like I just can't take it and I want to run out. I have always been a crier but being overwhelmed has never affected me this way before. In addition to anxiety, I am also experiencing vaginal dryness, hot flashes (a little bit), some hair thinning, forgetting how to do things that I have done for years plus some fogginess.

The forgetfulness is kind of scary. Some days I'm not able to do something that I have done for years. I can't remember how. So I'll just sit and ponder until it comes back to me and most of the time it does.

About 2-3 years ago, I had an embarrassing moment. One day at work, I volunteered to go out and get our lunches. It was no big deal because there was this little restaurant nearby, but I could not find the street. It was a street that I had driven hundreds of times. That was really scary. I don't know if I kept passing by it or what, but I could not find it. I just drove around for hours until I finally found it. I never told anyone about this before now.

Also, earlier in my childbearing years I had a tumor and had to have a hysterectomy. My husband was very angry with me because we could not have more children. But, I was very happy that I would no longer have a menstrual period.

I was married to a man who I felt was never in love with me. Everyone's needs always came before mine. So, when he came to me and said he wanted a divorce, I was devastated, it broke my heart. I cried every day for a year. I cried while on my way to work. I cried at work. I cried on my way home from work. It's still painful.

43

We had been married 25 years and I see all my friends who are still married such as my girlfriend who married about a year before we did and is celebrating 38 years of marriage. I loved being married, I loved being a wife and it still hurts my heart to think about it.

I met someone who was going through the same thing I was going through and he treated me like a queen. He was pressuring me to get married right away and I didn't feel that marriage was the right thing at the time. We both were just getting over hurt and pain of another relationship and I believed we couldn't be healed by marriage. Consequently we drifted apart, and then he got very sick and has since passed away. I still mourn for him because he treated me so well.

I am now in a long distance relationship that really isn't serious. I believe I deserve more. I have prayed for the Lord to send me someone, because I don't want to go through this life by myself, I want to have a mate.

❖ **Dry eyes** - Your eyes tend to be dry and itchy often – As a result of your eyes being dry they have a propensity to water easily. Your eyes are trying to compensate for the dryness which causes the tearing. Be sure to see your optometrist for an exam, prescription or suggestions on how to keep your eyes moistened. Keep in mind long term dryness if left untreated could cause some optical issues. Also, dry eyes may occur not only if you don't produce enough tears, but if you produce poor-quality tears.

Dry eyes feel uncomfortable, may sting or burn. You may experience dry eyes in certain situations, such as on an airplane, in an air-conditioned room or after looking at a computer screen for a few hours. When in a severe state or condition they are visibly red and tired looking.

Dry eye treatments can include lifestyle changes and eye drops. For more serious cases of dry eyes, surgery may be an option. [34]

Facial hair - Most women are not prepared for this symptom. It is when they experience hair popping out from under and around the jaw line, upper lip and neck area. This unpleasant, physical episode of unwanted facial hair occurs as a result of lower amounts of estrogen in the body and the testosterone (male hormones) becoming more dominate. Hairs begin to grow in the most precarious places. Per a fact provided by Holly Thacker, M.D. of Center for Specialized Women's Health. At age 55 men and women have the same amount of Estrogen in their bodies. This unwanted facial hair can be different for every woman, from a few hairs on the chin, light growth on the upper lip or heavy and beard like. To explain more in-depthly; when estrogen predominates, a woman's face typically has vellus hair –fine, short and almost invisible like 'peach fuzz'. Men, in contrast, have terminal hair, the longer, coarser, darker beard-type hair.

During reproductive years, the higher relative levels of estrogen to testosterone usually keep production of DHT

(Dihydrotesterone)low. However, as menopause approaches and estrogen levels drop, there's an increase of DHT in the hair follicle. It's at this point many women begin to see frustrating 'beard-like' hairs in places they've never seen them before, chin, jaw line, cheeks, and even the forehead.[35]

What should you do you may ask, and my answer is, to find a good pair of tweezers and begin plucking hairs out one by one or, you could wax them. There are creams available that can reduce the growth of facial hair. Find one that is FDA approved. Some women can take advantage of laser treatments, or remove hair from the roots with the use of a cotton thread by trained practitioners. Sorry, these are my only recommendations.

❖ **Craving of sugar and carbohydrates** - While you are really trying to watch your weight, you are being sabotaged by your own cravings. You crave simple carbohydrates more than usual. One of the reasons you are craving sugar is because of low adrenal function. The adrenals are hormone glands that sit above the kidneys. Amongst other things, one of their jobs is to secrete epinephrine (better known to some as adrenaline) which provides us with energy. Secondly, they secrete cortisone when there is inflammation present in the body. Thirdly, they replace the function of the ovaries in the production of the female hormones estrogen and progesterone when women get close to their menopausal years. When everything is functioning well and everything is being nourished properly, there is no problem.[35]

❖ **Urinary Tract Infections** - Women who have never had them before are now complaining about UTI's or bladder infections. The NIH (National Institute of Health) suggests urinary tract infections are caused by germs, usually bacteria that enter the urethra and then the bladder. This can lead to infection, most commonly in the bladder itself, which can spread to the kidneys.

Most of the time, your body can get rid of these bacteria. However, certain conditions increase the risk of having UTIs. Women tend to get them more often because their urethra is shorter and closer to the anus than in men. Because of this, women are more likely to get an infection after sexual activity or when using a diaphragm for birth control.

Menopause also increases the risk for UTI due to weakening (atrophy) of the vaginal walls. [37] This is primarily due to estrogen loss, which thins the walls of the urinary tract and reduces its ability to resist bacteria. [38]

It is recommended that women see their physicians, but in the meantime, you can drink water, approximately 6-8 glasses per day and lots of cranberry juice to flush out the bacteria.

❖ **Weight gain**- Weight gain is a real issue for mid-life women. Nancy Dell, registered dietitian, talks about menopause and weight gain. She tells that we are all born with fat cells. Attached to the membrane of these cells is an enzyme known by the initials LPL (Lipoprotein lipase). The purpose of this enzyme is to pull fat out of the blood stream and put the fat into the cell. When that happens our fat cells get bigger and we gain weight. The female hormone estrogen, reduces the activity of this LPL fat storing enzyme. So in menopause when estrogen levels drop, the LPL fat-storing enzyme becomes more active and you store more fat. Because middle-aged metabolism is real slow, you have to work extra hard to lose pounds. It means doing more to burn those calories or you will store them. Unfortunately, those extra calories turn to fat. It has been said that women gain an average of 10 pounds per year.

That is why so many women have the spare tire around the middle that was once reserved for men, or in today's terms, the "muffin top". No matter what it is labeled, it is unwanted fat around the waist and stomach area. It's when your love handles burst out over the top of your tight pants, giving your lower back/butt the appearance of a muffin.[39]

As your lifestyle and weight management coach, I can provide you with valuable tips designed to promote weight loss. These items are simple and proven:

•   Practice portion control - Focus on having the right portion size of food in your plate. For example; half of your plate should have fresh vegetables(1-2 cups), fourth of your plate should have   protein (4-6 oz lean meat or ½ cup beans, etc) and the remaining fourth should have starches (½ cup). Use a 9 inch plate at every meal.

•   Make healthy choices - Every day, you have to make choices of what you will eat. I am suggesting that you make conscious, wise decisions when selecting each meal, selecting snacks and especially when eating out. When making those choices determine which foods will provide nutrients and lower calories.

•   Stop eating at the first sign of feeling full. Until your brain registers what that feels like, it will take some practice. Sometimes you need strength to push yourself away from the table. We are so used to feeling overly stuffed until we believe that that is normal. I am here to dispel that myth. Try this, practice eating slowly and when your stomach is beginning to feel full, put the fork or spoon down and wait. What is your brain telling you?

• Avoid simple carbohydrates - I am referring to refined carbohydrates, like white sugar and white flour. This list will include; cakes, cookies, pies, candy, white bread, white rice, white pastas and other starchy products. I really promote staying away from processed foods, shelf foods, packaged in boxes or bags.

• Steer clear of saturated and trans fats. Research shows bad fats increase your cholesterol and your risk of certain diseases, while good fats have the opposite effect, protecting your heart and supporting overall health. In fact, good fats — such as omega-3 fats — are absolutely essential not only to your physical health but your emotional well-being.[39]

• Drink lots of water. There are several schools of thought about water, but the simplest is drink 6- 8 (8oz) glasses of water every day. This helps to cleanse the body and wash away the fat. Note: The purpose is to keep the body hydrated inside and out, because a hydrated body is a healthy body.

"An archeologist is the best husband a woman can have: the older she gets, the more interested he is in her"- Agatha Christie, English writer (1890–1976)

Her Story 5 - Wendy

When I first started my symptoms at about age 48 yrs old, I did not believe I was in menopause. The only thing that convinced me was my irregular cycle. But, friends said I was moody and I know I was real tearful. Once the crying started I could not stop. I also had night sweats. Even now, I experience hot flashes.

When I go out, like shopping or to the restaurant, I must know where all the bathrooms are because I always have to go to the bathroom. Maybe I should put on Depends for leakage protection. Also I must remember to have a fan available because I might drip sweat when everyone else appears cool and comfortable. I feel kind of bad when everyone is looking at me. Another frustrating thing is my weight fluctuates. The fat stays around the belly and it does not want to leave. In the past I could drop 10 pounds in 2 weeks. Now, it takes about 2 months to drop 10 pounds.

I believe (and I accept) that I am finally in the menopausal stage. My understanding is if I have not had a menstrual cycle for at least a year, I am in menopause. Well, I have not had a period for 15 months, so I think I have made it.

Menopause is just a part of life. It is just a phase of puberty, just the old phase. Yes, I am a little bit in denial. I choose not to speak it out loud. Really, I am proud to be in the class of menopausal ladies. At this age, a mature age, you should be able to say what you want to say and do what you want to do and not care about what others think about you, I think I am there.

I don't believe I focus on menopause because I have so much going on in my life. First of all, I had my children late in life. At age 30, I had my first born and age 35 my second child. So, I have children at home. My husband passed four years ago. My mother (who needs total care) moved in with me about two years ago so I am a care giver. This leaves little to no time to focus on my issues.

(IN THE MIDDLE OF THE INTERVIEW SHE BEGAN SWEATING)

My friends are younger than me, but slowly approaching age 50. I am so excited they will be joining me. Right now, they talk about me and joke about my hot flashes, but in a few years they will all be sweating with me. When they begin, it is possible I will be finished with that phase.

I don't know if this is a symptom of menopause, but I tend to forget a lot more. Sometimes, when I leave home I cannot remember if I turned the appliances off. I misplace my keys all the time, so now I have a special place for them right at the door.

Many times I carry two purses. I put a purse inside of a purse to keep myself organized. The purpose is to make sure I don't forget anything important that I use every day, so those items remain inside the inner purse. Subsequently, if I change outer purses I will still have everything I need inside the inner purse. It makes sense to me. It's one of my tricks to accommodate my forgetfulness.

My advice to other women is to ride the wave, because this will pass, but if you cannot endure, seek help from a doctor or herbalist or whomever you feel comfortable with... Don't be afraid to ask for help.

I believe we need to educate our young women about the sexual aspect or they will not be prepared. When in their 20's-30's it's about getting it on, but as women get older their priorities become raising children, working, and paying bills. Plus, women are usually tired, sweaty and don't want to be bothered. Men need to understand it is not about them. Women don't want to be like that but, they can't help it. My understanding is that later on in life sexual libido comes back. It goes away but eventually, it will be okay.

<u>Inserted 4 weeks after the initial interview</u>: "Oh no, I do not believe this is happening! I am having a period after 15 months. It has been recommended that I see my doctor to make sure all is well, but does this mean I have to start counting all over again?"

CHAPTER 4

HOTFLASHES - IS IT HOT IN HERE OR IS IT ME?

Her Story 6 – Linda (Me)

On September 11, 2001, everything changed for the United States of America, and it also changed for me. I, along with a friend, a fellow employee, was attending the last day of the Annual Candy Show in King Of Prussia, Pennsylvania, 20 miles from Philadelphia at a Convention Center. We both began hearing talks around the Convention Center that a plane had flown into one of the Twin Towers in New York City. I immediately went to the information counter to ask about what was going on. Luckily, they were watching TV and I saw, first hand, the second plane as it flew into the second tower, followed by the plane that had hit the Pentagon and the fourth one which crashed in Pennsylvania. I knew immediately we were not going anywhere any time soon. I asked the front desk if I could use the telephone and made reservations at a hotel for my friend and me. We stayed tuned to the TV to find out what our fate would be for the next several days in Pennsylvania. Well, no planes, trains, buses or cars were leaving Philadelphia and we were stuck. We were there 4 days and that is when they began…

I was sitting on the bed reading some material I had obtained from the candy show, when all of a sudden, this intense surge of heat began to move up my body. Slowly, but powerfully, the heat starting around my waist area and by the time it reached my face, I was anxious, hot, and sweaty.

I told my friend what I had just experienced and she told me that I was having hot flashes. Mind you, I was 48 and had never thought about hot flashes so, this was a foreign concept to me. But that evening, I became very familiar with them because they continued all night long, which resulted in us turning on the air conditioning so I could get some relief. That was the first time I slept all night - with air conditioning. Because my friend was older than I, this was not unusual for her and she was comfortable with the air conditioning. More than 6-8 months passed before I experienced another episode of hot flashes.

This is my favorite topic. I realize that is an oxymoron, but because so many people outwardly experience this symptom it appears to be the most "in your face" symptom of all of them. Even though it may be the most observed and openly discussed symptom, it is by no means the most important.

When I see a fellow menopausal woman sweating, I feel a sense of sisterhood, or empathy, because I understand what she is going through and I can relate to her discomfort and plight. I want to say, "It's okay girl. I go through the same thing. Or, I see you are experiencing your own personal summer", just anything to provide some level of comfort for her and maybe even open it up for discussion. Or, better yet, "Yes, Real Women Do Sweat".

Because I have studied hot flashes for several years, I have been able to develop a list of potential and proven remedies that seem to be common among researchers that can help the average woman. Just like anything else, every remedy will not work on every woman. You can only find out through trial and error. Just a word of caution, whatever you do, don't try to ignore your hot flashes in hopes that they go away. Become proactive and do something that will improve your quality of life.

What are Hot flashes?

Believe me, if you are experiencing them, you already know what they feel like, but my goal is to educate women so they understand them. According to *Menopause for Dummies,* "Hot flashes occur when the brain's temperature mechanism, the hypothalamus, is malfunctioning. It sometimes sends a message to the brain that the body is cool or hot so the brain sends messages through the body particularly the blood vessels to heat the body up even though the person may currently be comfortable or it might try to cool them down. When that erroneous message is sent the body heats up and hence, hot flashes.[40] Here are a few common characteristics: they tend to last between 30 seconds and 6 minutes, they could occur once a day or once every hour of the day, one may experience night sweats in addition to daytime hot flashes and the upper body is more likely to heat up.

However, what many women do not realize is there are <u>controllable</u> triggers that bring on most hot flashes and night sweats, which was discussed earlier. It is extremely important to identify what those triggers are. Here is a list of a few common ones that most women are affected by: soda pop, caffeine, alcohol, salt, hot or spicy foods, chocolate, hot drinks, sugary beverages, hot environments, sugary foods, artificial sweeteners, anxiety or stress, and especially cigarette smoking. A study was published in the *National Association of Menopause(NAM)-Obstet Gynecol* magazine in 2008 indicating that among women who smoke cigarettes endure hot flashes at a higher rate in midlife than non-smoking women.[42]

Indeed, identifying triggers is an extremely important first step towards determining the lifestyle changes that are necessary in order to live a gratifying and healthier life. If you determine that eating chocolate candy or drinking coffee produces hot flashes you know these are items you must either reduce or totally eliminate from your diet.

For your entertainment I have listed my triggers that induce hot flashes:

I.   Chocolate- I love chocolate but the cocoa affects me adversely

II. Sugar- If I eat cake, candy, cookies or any product high in sugar usually 13 grams or higher

III. Caffeine-I do not drink coffee, but a cup of tea or hot chocolate or chocolate candy with caffeine

IV. Spicy foods- Any item that has or resembles peppers whether mild or hot

V.   Beef- hamburgers, steaks, sliced beef from briquettes (hormones in the animal)

VI. Anxiety-It has to be something that catches me unaware because by nature I am a cool, calm and collective person. I get anxious when I am caught off guard.

VII. Hot or cold environment-The room temperature is too hot or cold for my comfort level.

VIII. Artificial sweeteners-I know if I drink a beverage with artificial sweeteners not only does it have an unpleasant taste to me, but I also break out in a sweat immediately.

Thank goodness it is a fairly short list, but I take this list seriously. Use yours as a guide to determine what foods are troublesome for you, because they either cause you to feel or behave badly. Once you take some of these foods out of your diet or eat them sparingly, you will see a difference in how you feel and the number of hot flashes you experience. Once you have some control over the triggers, then, and only then, will you be on the road to living a quality life. This book will show women how to live with menopause and enjoy life. To decrease the number of hot flashes you experience each day is huge. You will feel like you are on the path to recovery while getting closer to normalcy again. Keep in mind even though the hot flashes are decreasing there are still other symptoms that need to be addressed.

Note: This portion of the book provides solutions to combating hot flashes. If you try something for a reasonable amount of time and it doesn't work for you, try something else. Keep experimenting until you find relief.

Two natural Hot flashes relievers are; Phytoestrogen foods and Exercise:

Phytoestrogen foods - There is growing evidence that eating foods rich in Phytoestrogen, plant substance that have an estrogen like activity, can be a significant help in easing hot flashes. Phytoestrogen are plants that produce their own estrogens that can be substituted for the estrogen our bodies no longer manufacture. Although they are weaker than natural estrogen they still have the ability to bind to estrogen receptors sites and when these sites receive the proper amount of estrogen stimulation, we feel great. But when they don't, well that's when menopausal related symptoms like hot flashes take hold. An estrogen receptor is a protein molecule found inside those cells that are targets for estrogen action. Estrogen receptors contain a specific site to which only estrogens (or closely related molecules) can bind.[43]

Examples of foods which are rich in Phytoestrogen:

• Omega 3 which is found in flaxseeds, almonds and salmon
• Fruits and vegetables-apples, cherries, olives, plums, broccoli,cauliflower, brussel sprouts, cabbage, egg plant,

tomatoes, garlic, onions, potatoes, alfalfa sprouts, peppers, chili, carrots, and yams;
- Beans, grains & seeds, peanuts, soy products, peas, garbanzo beans, brown rice, bulgur, oats, wheat germ and rye.
- Soy plants contain 3 of the most potent Phytoestrogen available –genistun, daizein and glycitein. They fall under a category known as isoflavones. You can find soy in, tofu, tempeh, soymilk, soy yogurt, meso, edamame, flaxseed, soynuts, soy protein drinks, etc.

Exercise to decrease the intensity of hot flashes. There is no substitute for exercising. For some this is the most difficult course of action to take towards wellness. We tend to find every excuse there is, from; there isn't enough time to we are just too tired, but the benefits outweigh the excuses. Benefits such as, reduction of blood pressure, and risk for cardiovascular diseases, strengthening of bones, reducing osteoporosis, increasing energy and promoting sleep. Exercising biologically releases natural endorphins that give you the feeling of well-being, or just feeling good. It is recommended that you exercise at least 4-5 times every week for 45 minutes to 1 hour. If you need to be around people and have structure, you can join your local gym, YMCA or recreation center. I always remind my clients that the great thing about exercising is you can do it free. You can walk, hike, run, or engage in other great outdoor activities, which leaves you with no excuse.

Be creative with your exercising. If you are not normally an outdoors person, get out and become one with nature. Explore, smell the flowers, watch the beautiful birds, take the dog (if you have one) down a trail and really observe and listen to the sounds. Get out and soak in the sun. Many people have exercise DVD's which allows them to exercise in the comfort of their own homes in front of the TV. Remember, there is no good excuse not to exercise.

"Freedom is doing what we like. Happiness is liking what you do." Unknown author

The Art of Journaling

This is a technique that I've adopted in my weight loss clubs, one on one coaching sessions and group presentations, and I use it to track my own hot flashes. It really works, so I subsequently recommended it to all of the women I speak with. My belief is, it is important to track your journey while you are going through menopause.

This technique is so valuable, ultimately, it allows you the ability to see the pattern developing in your experiences. Once you can see that pattern, you can begin to make changes. For example, if you realize after eating spicy foods you have a series of hot flashes then you know that you have to either eat those foods in moderation or stay completely away from them. Think about how empowering this is. You are more in control of your experiences. You will be able to predict your hot flashes, decrease their occurrences and even handle them better because they are not as evasive or unpredictable as before. When you believe you are more in control, you are less anxious about menopause as a whole and definitely better equipped to handle hot flashes.

How to Journal

1. Select a blank book you can carry around. It should be small enough to carry in a purse or business brief case.
2. Begin a list with the following headings: Breakfast, Lunch, Snack, and Dinner and after each item you ate indicate whether or not you experienced hot flashes and the level of intensity and for how long.
3. Reflections -Write about your experiences, feelings and any revelations that could assist you on this journey

---

4.   Explanation-Write down every single morsel or beverage that you put into your mouth-I recommend you do this for 30 days. After that time you will see a pattern. Map out that pattern so you have a clear understanding about which foods and beverages trigger your hot flashes.

Two Examples of Reflections

1. *"After reading my journal entries I noticed that I had 4 cups of coffee today, and three of them were before lunchtime. No wonder the hot flashes were so severe this morning. I am going to make an attempt to drink more water and less coffee. But, how can I stay alert all day. I need something to keep me stimulated."*

One other section you can include is the anxiety or stress piece. Stress also brings about hot flashes. Write down anything that is stressing you out that day and how often you are having hot flashes:

2. *"Today I was told by my supervisor he is unable to attend a very important meeting and that I must prepare to give a presentation that is due by 8:00 a.m. I have been experiencing hot flashes all day long. Is there any relief?"*

This reflection indicates that you are "under the gun" and extremely stressed about making a presentation for your supervisor and consequently you are experiencing continuous hot flashes resulting from some anxiety.

Note: On the next page, you will find a sample chart. Use the chart to help track your hot flashes and triggers. There is also a blank chart at the back of this book for your convenience with getting started.

Sample Chart

Breakfast 8:30 a.m.	Bowl of cereal	2% milk	1 pastry (Hot flashes, but not very intense)	
Snack	Spicy chicken sandwich-Hot flashes(intense, perspired a little)	2 Cups of coffee-Hot flashes-(very intense)		
Lunch	Spicy bean Chili-Hot flashes (Very intense-Perspired a lot. Hot flashes continued all afternoon.)	Crackers	Can of soda pop	
Snack	Chocolate candy bar-hot flashes (barely there)			
Dinner	Chicken-baked	Vegetable	Potatoes-baked	Pepsi-Hot flashes(perspired a little)
Snack Before Bed	Cup of coffee	Chocolate chip cookies – Night sweats intense - perspired a lot!		

Her Story 7 – Marie

I was in my early 40's when my menstrual periods took on noticeable changes. I was skipping, spotting for periods of 30 days, longer and heavier and that was a distressing time for me. I would always be tired, moody and cranky. My father use to say to me, "Do you have one good week out of the month?"

Leading into Menopause I began to keep a calendar to mark my cycles. I would have further stretches between cycles and I rejoiced. Then, when I turned 50 and had blood work done it was confirmed I was officially menopausal. On my calendar I put exclamation marks on that date. I was so looking forward to it. And when I shared my positive feelings with women they were always so negative. But, I decided I was going to treat it with my reality and not other people's reality. For me, I no longer had to think about getting pregnant. I never wanted to have children so the end of my period did not mean I missed the opportunity to have a family. The irony was my libido went south. Along with it went sexual feelings and energy. To this day, I am still going through it and at times I miss that feeling. Sometimes, it drove my behaviors, but the liberating thing is now my choices in life are driven more from my head versus from my physical needs.

I have educated myself to understand what I am going through. I read and research and have joined a blogging group. But I still try to accept my truth and not theirs. Initially, hot flashes were very disconcerting and embarrassing for me. They are not too bad now. But, not long ago I was in a store shopping and both hot flashes and anxiety hit at the same time and I had to leave the store. The good thing is, I saved myself money that day.

Now, I can have hot flashes in my office or around people and I make light reference to them until I am finished sweating. I am no longer embarrassed.

I notice I get more teary-eyed than I use to, but I am not sure if that is because of menopause or turning age 50. Either way, there is some grieving going on. For me it's about letting go of any belief that I am young. In my 40's I was very sexual, I looked young, even though I look good now, but no denying, I am moving past middle age. I'm dealing with one day I will no longer be around. I do a lot of reflecting now. I feel more fragile and sensitive.

There is something about whether I still have the "It factor". Am I still attractive, vital, and sexual? I didn't realize those things were important to me, to still feel attractive, sexy and feel like a woman. What I am finding is – Yes, you can still have "It" at 50.

Some days I do not want attention. But, I still get it even from younger guys. Sometimes that throws me. It's a different kind of beauty that comes from inside. So, what we do not have in looks, other things such as energy, maturity or self understanding make up for it.

Too many believe that their periods represent who they are as a woman. That is not what makes a woman. Having children does not make a woman. Society has defined us as; we must have babies, we must have sex, and we have to have a man. I don't see those things as defining me, but some women do.

I do not plan to do hormone treatment. My mother had breast cancer at age 53 and she took estrogen for perimenopause and she had a hysterectomy at age 42. Most of my readings connect HT with breast cancer. Not all, but, I made a conscious decision age 35 I was not going to use hormones. It is not for me.

CHAPTER 5

ACCEPTANCE OF MENOPAUSE FROM COCOON TO BUTTERFLY

Approaching menopause as a midlife transition engenders a sense of control and empowerment while setting a positive stage for the next trimester of life. [44]

Indeed, I believe there is a science to accepting menopause since it is not a simple time in our lives. From the beginning of puberty girls had to deal with menstrual periods for approximately 40 years and the majority of us couldn't wait until that stage of our lives was over.

Most of us were probably looking forward to the time when we would no longer have menstrual periods or PMS, only to discover that menopause can be just as difficult to deal with. That is why it is imperative to accept menopause as your new norm, be optimistic and accepting.

I know you are questioning whether you can live through this. Sure, you can. You are not dying, you are going through menopause. You can either, give up and be miserable, complain, or you can learn how to live with it, even find contentment in it. Picture a greenish yellow, creepy crawler, the caterpillar, one of God's strangest looking specimens. She transforms from a larvae through metamorphosis to a pupa. The pupa then builds her cocoon.

This complete metamorphosis literally means changing from one creature into a completely different creature.

When she emerges from the cocoon, she is a beautiful, colorful butterfly or moth. The length of this process, depends on the species and the season, could take a few weeks to several months. This is where I want you to use your imagination and correlate yourself with a butterfly.

The perimenopause phase is the caterpillar (creepy and crawly), the menopausal phase is the cocoon (even though you might be in there for years), and post menopausal is where you emerge into a beautiful butterfly.

Here, you've made a complete metamorphosis. All of the negative thoughts you have had about yourself and menopause has to be changed. Remember it is defined as, literally changing from one creature to a completely different one.

Change can be scary and I don't recommend that you go through this process alone. Surround yourself with people who love you or even consider joining a support group (this is discussed later in the book). It's rather therapeutic communing with other women who have or are currently going through the same experiences and to find out what remedies may have worked for them to relieve some of their symptoms.

The best advice I can offer to you is to become educated, read, study and do research to learn everything you can about perimenopause, menopause, and post menopause. This recommendation is repeated numerous times throughout the book. My philosophy is if life doesn't catch you off guard or if there are no surprises you can handle it better. Don't just let life happen to you. Make it happen for you.

Very briefly I want to address the emotional aspects of menopause. There are several dynamics in play when you are at the end of child bearing years, or youthful looks are fleeting or physical attractiveness becomes an issue. Additionally, you no longer feel comfortable in your skin and you no longer know your purpose in life.

One contextual factor, having multiple roles, has the potential to enhance women's adaptation to menopause. According to role-enhancement theory (Thoits, 1983), multiple roles can promote woman's development by increasing self-esteem, providing purpose and meaning in life, increasing one's ability to develop deep connections with others, and buffering against strain or difficulties experienced in one role. Paid work maybe particularly important as a buffer against loss of fertility during menopause, as work can provide women with a meaningful identity that is not rooted in their capacity to carry children. The first factor reflects attitudes pertaining to loss of childbearing capacity, as reflected in concerns about loss of fertility and affective response to the last period. The second factor reflects concerns about changes in health and physical attractiveness.[45]

In 2005 a study was presented by Shirley B. Huffman, Jane E. Myers, and Lloyd Bond, Focusing on Menopause and African-American Women: Attitudes and Symptom Reporting stated: "The picture of midlife African American women that emerged from this study supports a multicultural perspective that postmenopausal women recorded the most positive attitudes. Taken as a whole, women in this study reported a slightly positive attitude toward menopause, although they held many negative beliefs about it. They believed menopause is both a natural midlife event and a reason to seek medical attention. Forty-nine percent believed women worry about losing their minds during menopause, while 71% believed women are concerned about how their husbands will feel about them after menopause. On the other hand, they believed after menopause women have a broader outlook on life and generally feel better than they have for years."[45] (*Managing Menopause Naturally*)

As women, we spend every waking hour helping

and serving others and seldom do we focus on ourselves. Remember how I said it is important to reinvent yourself? Well, this is the time to engage in activities that you really enjoy. Think of all the things that make you happy. Make a list of those things that make you happy and all the new things you want to bring into your life. Develop your "Bucket List".

The more you seek pleasure, the more pleasure will find you. Ask yourself when was the last time you did something for yourself like getting a manicure or pedicure. Take dancing or golfing lessons, run a marathon, or at least train for it, and even take piano lessons at your age.

I had a very good friend who bought a brand new piano, took lessons for a year, and invited her friends over for a recital. We had a wonderful time.

You can do whatever you put your mind to doing. In fact, you are limited only by your own mind. If you allow yourself to think big you will do big things and visa versa. By doing nothing, you will wither away. Don't let that happen. Spread out your beautiful butterfly wings today and fly.

Something for the soul; "Fear less, hope more, whine less, breathe more; talk less, say more, hate less, lose more and all good things are yours" - Anonymous

CHAPTER 6

SUPER FOODS–PHYTOESTROGEN FOR THE SUPER WOMAN

Essentially, there are foods that are considered to be lifesavers. Each nutritionist has a list of favorite "super foods." Each of them recommend that you make these foods part of your daily eating plan to ensure a quality of life. The important aspect of these lists is the foods that are on the lists are designed to provide substance needed for the majority of menopausal symptoms.

To build a healthy body, these foods are crucial. The foods provide you with necessary vitamins and minerals the body needs to look good and feel good. According to *Menopause for Dummies*, below are 10 power foods and how they benefit the body:

1. **Soy**-Doctors agree one serving a day is safe and decreases hot flashes
2. **Nuts**–walnuts and almonds contain linoleic, alpha-linoleic fatty acids, antioxidants, magnesium, Vitamin. E, sedemium and other nutrients
3. **Salmon**-for Omega 3 and protein. Salmon decrease osteoporosis, blood clots, and some cancers
4. **Yams**-antioxidant, potassium, Vitamin C, magnesium, Bit B6, and fiber
5. **Berries** -blue, raspberry or strawberries for antioxidants, Vitamin C

6. **Flax seeds**-meal or oil (more affective) for heart and hot flashes
7. **Oranges**-Vitamin C, antioxidants, lower risk of stomach cancer
8. **Teas**-black & green are powerful antioxidant polyphenos, which makes them affective at fighting cell damage associated with inflammation and heart disease.
9. **Green vegetables**-leafy green vegetables. The less cooked the better
10. **Yogurt**-In addition to dairy low fat yogurt, soy yogurt is beneficial - great source of calcium[47]

Per Dr. David Heber, author of *What Color Is Your Diet?: Color Code Foods Made Easy,* (pg. 44), he defined this group of foods as valuable because of the vitamins and minerals received when consumed: It is amazing all of the beautiful bountiful colors nature provides for us and how each color represents nutrition. This color code system is so easy it can be used by the entire family. If you are sincerely interested in living a healthy lifestyle, just follow his recommendation and you are sure to see some improvement.

Breakdown by color code

1. **Red group**: canned or bottled tomato juice a mixed vegetable juice; canned tomatoes, tomato paste tomato sauce, pasta sauces; prepared tomato soup; prepared tomato salsa; chilled, pre-sliced pink grapefruit; precut watermelon in season
2. **Red/purple group**: Bottle grape juice (100 percent juice), bottled cranberry juice or frozen cranberry juice concentrate, frozen whole berries, pre-shredded purple cabbage, cooked or for slaws, frozen sliced peppers, and fresh apples, pears, berries, and cherries.

3. **Orange group:** Prewashed and cut or shredded carrots, frozen carrots, and frozen winter squash; pre-sliced mango available fresh-chilled or packed in juice or as frozen mango chunks; precut cantaloupe wedges or balls; and whole fresh apricots.

4. **Orange/yellow group**: Fresh orange juice, frozen orange juice or tangerine juice concentrate; pre-sliced papaya, pineapple, and yellow grapefruit sections available fresh or chilled and packed in juice; frozen pineapple chunks; pineapple canned in pineapple juice; fresh whole nectarines, oranges, peaches, and tangerines.

5. **Yellow/green group:** Fresh or frozen spinach, collard greens, mustard greens, avocados, and turnip greens. Loose-pack spinach in bags is particularly convenient because you can add only what you need to soups, mixed dishes, omelets, and pasta. Frozen pepper slices are easily added to dishes, and pre-washed salad greens and raw spinach made quick work of a colorful salad. Look for precut honeydew melon.

6. **Green group**: Pre-washed-and-cut broccoli florets and broccoli stems for slaw, and broccoli sprouts, make getting these healthy vegetables much easier. Pre-shredded cabbage for cooking or for slaw, pre-washed-and-cut cauliflower florets, and frozen broccoli and cauliflower are also widely available.

7. **White/green group:** If you don't like preparing onions and garlic, you can find pre-chopped garlic in jars and packaged, pre-chopped fresh onion in the produce section. Washed and sliced celery stalks are great for snacking, and sliced mushrooms are available packaged and at many supermarket salad bars.[47]

I have always been extremely fascinated with the Asian traditional diet which is extremely healthy when prepared in a traditional manner. Asian woman eat healthier foods and according to some studies have fewer menopausal symptoms.   For example, their daily diet consist of rice, whole grains, whole grain breads, noodles, millet, corn, vegetables, fruits and legumes (beans), fish, shellfish and dairy optional daily and eggs and poultry, weekly, sweets weekly and meats especially red, monthly.

Around 2000, the Asian Pyramid was created by Cornell China, Oxford Project on Nutrition, and it was very different from the USDA Pyramid.   The Asian Pyramid promoted grains and vegetables as the diets staple and should be eaten everyday several times a day. According to that Pyramid meat is eaten sparsely (monthly) with desserts weekly and wine and beer in moderation.

Her Story 8 – Audie

I started menopausal symptoms about age 45. I am currently in the postmenopausal stage, so it was about 20 years ago.

My first symptom was irregular periods. I thought I was pregnant again. I also had hot flashes, night sweats, sleep interruptions, vaginal dryness and irritation, and I was short tempered. I had the type of night sweats that caused me to lose sleep at night, which increased my irritability. Then, I had to get up very early to go to work after getting a minimum amount of sleep and I was working with small children so that was not a very good combination.

I didn't know what was wrong with me; I just knew this was not normal. So, I went to see a doctor and he informed me it was perimenopause and suggested I use HRT. After several more nights of broken sleep and waking up soaked and wet, I started the Estrogen pills, which I took for several years. I wasn't happy with the pills, so I then went to a female doctor who suggested I stop taking them and try dealing with the menopause naturally and that is what I did. She recommended natural herbs and advised me to eat yams. For the vaginal dryness, she said I should try olive oil. I have to say the hot flashes came back when I stopped using HRT, but they did not last long.

My experiences affected my family in different ways. I was an older mother with a baby and I was very impatient with her. At the same time, I had an adult son who was driving me crazy because he was still at home and dependent and I had no patience for him. On the flip side, my husband was not really aware of my episodes. The only thing that affected him was when my night sweats began and I had to cool myself down. I needed to take the covers off or quickly figure out how to cool myself down. I tried to spare him as much as possible even though we did discuss it, and I would share written materials with him to educate him about what I was experiencing.

I also had to educate my students by default. I was a teacher and one day, I had an embarrassing moment at school. We had an emergency button in each classroom that anyone could

71

push in case of an emergency. So, one day I broke out into sweating profusely and the children were convinced that I was sick even though I tried to explain to them that I was okay. Well, one of the children pushed the emergency button which goes directly to the Principal's office. Someone rushed down to see what was going on in my classroom and I had to explain that I was just having hot flashes and there was no emergency.

Years ago, I used to sew all the time. It was my favorite hobby. I made all my baby's clothes. I was creative and I loved it. As she got older, I designed and sewed her school clothes as well. Then, when perimenopause hit, I could not stand to follow all the steps it took to sew. I would get so irritated at the smallest things and I could not fight through it. I had no patience. Then, it became a battle keeping my sewing scissors in my sewing room because my family members would use them and misplace them. I would spend so much time looking for the scissors that by the time I found them I no longer had the desire to sew. Because nothing seemed to go right, one day I packed up my sewing machine, tools, material and everything related to sewing and put them away. Now, after 20 years I have unpacked my sewing machine and I am starting to sew again.

I found the things I was experiencing through menopause, my closest friends were too young to understand and my older relatives chose not to talk about, so I had no one to discuss my issues with.

My recommendations are; 1. Be kind to yourself understand it is a part of a natural process and do things for yourself to feel better 2. Understand someday you will be happy and some days you may feel crazy, and 3. Try to share menopause issues with your mate so he can understand you better.

CHAPTER 7

ALTERNATIVE MEDICINE -SUPPLEMENTS/HERBS AND VITAMINS AND MINERALS

Vitamins are a vital part of my life. I learned years ago that it is not possible to consume all the vitamins or minerals our body needs to be well, feel well, or to provide the raw materials the body needs to heal itself by only consuming fruits, vegetables, grains, etc. that are purchased routinely from the grocery store.

Unfortunately, food no longer contains the amount of vitamins and minerals they did many years ago before pesticides and insecticides and genetic engineering became a part of the planting and growing process.

Today, the soil is undernourished and contaminated. As a result you would have an extremely difficult time getting the recommended daily allowance of vitamins and minerals your body needs, unless you are fortunate enough to purchase year round from a local farmer. Subsequently, supplements are critical.

If you are not a current vitamin taker, when you do start you will notice the transformation almost immediately. You will feel different, more invigorated, have more energy, may even sleep better. Also, your skin, eyes, finger nails, and hair will begin to look better. I have been taking them for over 38 years and if I compare my body, health, and appearance to others my age there is a major difference.

I don't have heart problems, cholesterol problems, diabetes problems, etc., etc., etc. Just because you are getting older chronologically does not mean your body has to age at the same speed. When you are rebuilding those cells it is almost like turning back the clock or at least slowing it down.

I have always bought my products from either health food stores or ordered them direct from companies. These companies through proven research and development, manufactures products that are safe for human consumption and the environment. They use natural versus man-made ingredients to develop a natural product. All vitamins are not created equal. Let me repeat myself. All vitamins are not created equal. Many of the popular, commercial brands are not the healthiest brands.

Natural vs. Manmade - If you study vitamins, you will find that some vitamins obtain majority of their ingredients from nature, and have little to no byproducts, fillers or any unnecessary ingredients. To this end they will have a more positive effect on the body, are safer, healthier and do not cause side effects. Simply explained, manmade vitamins are manufactured by using synthetic ingredients for the substances and also use synthetic ingredients to create the pill coating, which make a difference when you swallow them.

Over three decades, I have tried many different types of vitamins and minerals manufactured by many different companies. What I took depended on what my needs were at the time or what phase of my life I was in. Today is no different, I am taking vitamins dictated by the phase of my life I am in now. I have selected these particular ones to share to provide a model for you the reader. Once again you will need to read and study the ends and outs of vitamins and minerals for yourself to determine which nutrients are best for you to take daily. But this is what I currently take and why;

1) Multivitamins with Minerals for women over 50 which contains the following: Vitamins A, C,E, B12,Zinc, Copper, Riboflavin, Thiamin-to provide the foundation necessary to keep the body's cells rejuvenating. Find a multivitamin that contains what you need.

2) Calcium with Vitamin D. Everyone needs calcium and Vitamin D and it has been proven they work better when taken together. I take recommended amounts for women over 50; Calcium 1500mg and 1000IU of Vit D. Know that your calcium is decreasing daily and if not replaced, you'll have to contend with Osteoporosis and/or low bone density. Vitamin D promotes calcium absorption in the gut and maintains adequate serum calcium and phosphate concentrations to enable normal mineralization of bone and to prevent hypocalcemic tetany. Without sufficient vitamin D, bones can become thin, brittle, or misshapen.[49]

3) An Immune building system. Vitamins which include; Echinacea, Vitamin C, Zinc and Vitamin E to ward off common colds.

4) Estrogen replacement vitamins-There are several companies that produce natural herbal vitamins that can be obtained from the local health food store to handle or manage your menopause symptoms. One capsules contains: Dried Soy Extract, Dried Dong Quai Extract, Dried Black Cohosh (It works for me)

5) Vitamin B12- as stress reliever-Vitamin B12 is a nutrient that helps keep the body's nerve and blood cells healthy and helps make DNA, the genetic material in all cells. Vitamin B12 also helps prevent a type of anemia called megaloblastic anemia that makes people tired and weak.[50]

6) Omega 3 and fish oil –This is an essential fat because our body does not produce it and healthy fats are necessary.There is evidence from multiple studies supporting intake of recommended amounts of DHA and EPA in the form of dietary fish or fish oil supplements lowers triglycerides, reduces the risk of death, heart attack, dangerous abnormal heart rhythms, and strokes in people with known cardiovascular disease, slows the buildup of atherosclerotic plaques ("hardening of the arteries"), and lowers blood pressure slightly.[51]

In addition to vitamins, herbs have proven to be a popular substance with those who practice holistic medicine, so I will highlight just a few well known herbs. Many of these herbs work the same as phytoestrogens. They serve as weak substitutes for our estrogen and individuals who choose to use herbs to deal with menopausal symptoms have found profound relief. While researching relief tactics, I found herbs that were mentioned many times as a form of natural treatment. Let's see what nature offers us:

1. Black Cohosh- Native Americans discovered that the root of the black cohosh plant (ACTAEA RACEMOSA, formerly known as CIMICIFUGA RACEMOSA) helped relieve menstrual cramps and symptoms of menopause,... Early German studies found black cohosh improved physical and psychological menopausal symptoms, including anxiety, hot flashes, night sweats, and vaginal dryness. The American College of Obstetricians and Gynecologists supports short-term use of black cohosh - up to six months - for treating menopausal symptoms. [51] Soy products, which are high in estrogen-like activity. Genistein, one of soy's most active isoflavones, is found in many menopause supplements. The large amount of tofu, soy milk, and

tempeh in the Japanese diet may be one reason why so few Japanese women report menopausal symptoms. In one study, post-menopausal women ate foods said to increase estrogen: soy, red clover sprouts, and flaxseeds.

2. Flaxseed, ground or oil- Early studies found that flax seeds may aid lowering total cholesterol and LDL cholesterol levels. They may also keep platelets from becoming sticky therefore reducing the risk of a heart attack. Aside from alpha linolenic acid, flaxseed is rich in lignan. Lignan is a type phytoestrogen (antioxidant) and also provides fiber. Researches revealed that lignan in flax seed shows a lot of promise in fighting disease -- including a possible role in cancer prevention especially breast cancer. It is thought that lignan metabolites can bind to estrogen receptors, hence inhibiting the onset of estrogen-stimulated breast.[52]

3. In extensive studies done in Europe, St. John's Wort has been shown to be highly effective in treating mild-to-moderate depression. Other supplements that have shown some success in treating menopause-related mood disorders include garden sage, ginseng, black cohosh, and dong quai.[53]

4. Dong Quai-It remains one of the most popular plants in Chinese medicine, and is used primarily for health conditions in women. Dong quai has been called "female ginseng," based on its use for gynecological disorders (such as painful menstruation or pelvic pain), recovery from childbirth or illness, and fatigue/low vitality. It is also given for strengthening *xue* (loosely translated as "the blood"), for cardiovascular conditions/high blood pressure, inflammation, headache, infections, and nerve pain. [54]

5. Valerian Root- Valerian herbal supplements   are widely used to combat sleeplessness, anxiety and stress. This all-natural remedy is derived from the valerian plant root and comes in many forms. Inconclusive

studies reported by the National Institutes of Health indicate valerian use, either in liquid form or in "commercial" supplements, improved the sleep quality and sleep latency in volunteers with mild insomnia. Valerian may be beneficial at helping you shorten the amount of time taken to fall asleep (sleep latency) and reducing instances of middle of the night wakefulness. [55] Each evening before you go to bed drink a cup of Valerian tea and enjoy a good nights' rest. But I must warn you that the Valerian tea has a strong, unpleasant, pungent odor

6. Ginkgo biloba extract is useful for the menopausal and postmenopausal woman because of its effects on the vascular system. It is especially useful in relieving both the cold hands and feet and the forgetfulness that often accompany menopause. Ginkgo biloba extract has also been shown to improve blood flow to the hands and feet in human clinical trials and has been shown to be effective in the treatment of peripheral vascular disease of the extremities. Ginkgo biloba extract has repeatedly been used to improve mental health in patients with cerebral vascular insufficiency and may exert similar effects in menopause. Ginkgo biloba extract appears to work not only by increasing blood flow to the brain, but also by enhancing energy production within the brain, increasing the uptake of glucose by brain cells and actually improving the transmission of nerve signals.[56]

We know that menopause has been around since the beginning of time, which leads me to believe that our women had solutions to deal with menopause way back then. I found out that there are several different home remedies that have been passed down from generation to generation by great-grandmothers, grandmothers, and some mothers. Maybe even you have heard of some of them. Be clear that I am not recommending any home remedies, but it was fascinating to me that they have been around for centuries and are still around in some medicine cabinets even today. For example, Lydia Pinkham, like many women of her time brewed home remedies, which she continually collected. Her remedy for "female complaints" became very popular among her neighbours to whom she gave it. Pinkham's solution was to mix vegetable roots with 19% alcohol.[57]

CHAPTER 8

HORMONE REPLACEMENT THERAPY

Up to this point in the book, I have discussed many different natural/holistic alternatives to being well. This chapter deals with finding relief using HT. The message I want to continuously convey is you must be proactive with menopause. There are techniques for quick or long term relief such as; taking vitamins, herbs, eating the power foods all the way to changing your lifestyle, or there is hormone replacement therapy, now referred to as hormone therapy.

Medical Dictionary's definition of hormone replacement therapy is, "involves the use of one or more of a group of medications designed to artificially boost hormone levels."

I am asked by many what my thoughts are on hormone replacement therapy or hormone therapy (HT). I have found several different studies that I will share and you can make up your own mind.

With anything, there are always pros and cons and you need to educate yourself to diligently weigh the two (Holistic vs. HT) to determine what is best for you. For example; Pros- it relieves menopausal symptoms. You enjoy a quality of life again immediately. You begin to feel normal again. The depression, mood swings, and anxiety go away and furthermore the hot flashes become controllable. You stop suffering from dry vaginal walls and most of all, you no longer feel like they are going out of your mind.

On the other hand, there are cons, particularly side effects. Researchers proved that certain kinds increased the risk for cancer, which is why it was taken off the market.

Several examples of side effects:

BLOOD CLOTS
Doctors have long known that taking estrogen increases a person's risk for blood clots. Generally, this risk is higher if you use birth control pills, which contain high doses of estrogen. Your risk is even higher if you smoke and take estrogen. The risk is not as high when estrogen skin patches (transdermal estrogen) are used.

CANCER
Breast cancer: Women who take estrogen therapy for a long period of time have a small increase in risk for breast cancer. Most guidelines currently consider hormone therapy safe for breast cancer risk when taken for up to 5 years. Endometrial/uterine cancer: The risk for endometrial cancer is more than five times higher in women who take estrogen therapy alone, compared with those who do not. However, taking progesterone with estrogen seems to protect against this cancer. Endometrial cancer does not develop in women who do not have a uterus. Long-term treatment with Premarin may increase your risk of breast cancer, heart attack, or stroke. Talk with your doctor about your individual risks before using Premarin long term, especially if you smoke or are overweight. Your doctor should check your progress on a regular basis (every 3 to 6 months) to determine whether you should continue this treatment.[58]

CARDIOVASCULAR DISEASE
Estrogen may increase the risk of heart disease in older women, or in women who began estrogen use more than 10 years after their last period. Estrogen is probably the safest when started in women under age 60, or within 10 years

after the start of menopause. As mentioned, women who take estrogen have an increased risk for stroke.

GALLBLADDER DISEASE

Several studies have shown that women who take estrogen/progestin therapy have an increased risk for developing gallstones.

In addition, some women taking hormone therapy may suffer from; bloating, breast soreness, headaches, mood swings, nausea, and water retention.

Some women have irregular bleeding when they start taking hormone therapy. Changing the dose often eliminates this side effect. Close follow-up with your doctor is important when you have any unusual bleeding.[60]

Note: Most women who take estrogen and who have not had their uterus removed also need to take progesterone. Taking these medicines together helps reduce the risk of endometrial (uterine) cancer. Continuous, combined therapy involves taking estrogen and progestin together every day. Irregular bleeding may occur when starting or switching to this therapy. Most women stop bleeding within 1 year.[61]

Another study was conducted by researcher Patrick Lefebvre, out of Montreal, Canada in 2011. His study consisted of 27,000 women who used trans dermal hormone replacement therapy (HRT) and 27,000 matched controls taking estrogen-only pills. Found that those who used estrogen patches were one-third less likely to develop deep vein thrombosis or pulmonary embolism. Past studies have found that hormone-patch users have a lower blood clot risk than women who take oral HRT containing both estrogen and progesterone Researchers think hormone patches may be less risky than pills because they bypass the liver and may not boost clot-promoting proteins in the blood.[62]

Vaginal Estrogen for vaginal dryness: There is one notable positive exception to usage of HT, that's prescriptions for topical (vaginal) estrogen products for menopausal use. Prescriptions for vaginal estrogens have raised steadily at the same time that prescriptions for HT products overall have fallen. According to the IMS National Prescription Audit Plus™, the number of prescriptions dispensed for vaginal estrogen products rose from 2.8 million in 2001 to 4.52 million in 2006 — a rise of 61% during these years when the use of systemic HT products fell sharply over safety concerns in the wake of the 2002 publication of initial results from the Women's Health Initiative trial. Dispensed prescriptions for vaginal estrogen products increased further from 4.52 million in 2006 to 5.29 million in 2010 — an increase of 17%. [62]

Her Story 9 – Dee

I started experiencing menopause around ages 46 or 47. Memory loss was my first symptom. Night sweats started for me within the last year. Vaginal dryness-last 2 years and my menstrual cycle has been different every month. Also, there is a level of confusion, such as my not just forgetting but not being able to grasp things that were once simple for me to do.

I am less patient with the simplest things. I used to be able to figure things out, but it's to the point where the frustration brings me to tears. When my husband needs information from me, I just want him to give me the bottom line and save his explanations. Usually, I am not on the same page anyway (Some things are too confusing). He is logical and balances everything to the penny but I'm not like that now.

Also, my taste for some foods has changed. For years I could not eat cherries and now I eat them. I heard your taste buds change with menopause.

During early menopause, I was frustrated with not being able to remember stuff, but I believe it was a result of getting older which I see as a blessing.

One of my forgetting stories is this: When I couldn't find my keys my husband was not happy about having to get up and help me look for them. We looked in the trash, refrigerator, underneath my car and the whole time they were in my pocket. I asked myself if I was losing my mind or going crazy. Then, I asked my husband and he said yes. And I just sat in my car and cried. I got to work and an older lady told me, no I am not going crazy. She said our minds are like computers that place information in files and stores it into compartments until we need it then it has to sort through all those files. Sometimes, it takes a while. It is very embarrassing to forget things in front of people stuff that you should know such as not being able spell words I have spelled all my life.

I am fairly a newlywed and I was excited and enthusiastic about sex. I thought it would be anywhere, anytime, but it did not happen that way. I am so glad I have an understanding husband, because there are times that I could care less, or it is uncomfortable or painful or frustrating because I have to go through so much preparation stuff whereas before things were lubricated naturally. I wish someone would have given me a heads-up on the sexual discomfort.

Yeast infections – Every other month for a week at a time, I get yeast infections and Vaseline comes to the rescue.

Also, now, I go to the bathroom a whole lot more. I drink a lot of water and I can't hold that water like I use to. So, I understand those commercials with the Depend products. I even use something just in case I have a leak. I never had to be concerned with that before.

My Recommendations are: Don't take menopause so seriously. I wish I had more funnies to talk about or even embarrassing moments, because I took it seriously. So, what is helping me out is to stop taking it so seriously. Now, I joke with my girlfriends about it and I talk to other women about it because I know I am not alone in this.

During this interview, I recognized the importance of sharing menopause with my daughter-in-law and I need to say something to other ladies I come in contact with that will be going through it also. "If you don't have a sense of humor you become a scowling time bomb, striking out a people who are dear to you". - Ishmael Reed

Linda Hawkins

CHAPTER 9

HOW MENOPAUSE AFFECTS THOSE YOU LOVE

There is no doubt that menopause affects every member of the household. The women's behavior, attitude and disposition affect those around her and usually those closest to her. If she is in a bad mood, that affects the family. If she suffers from anxiousness and experiences heart palpitations often, that affects the family. If her body temperature has gone array because of hot flashes and is in need of immediate relief, well, that could mean temporary or long term discomfort for the family, such as blasting the air conditioner or opening windows when the house may already be cold. If she is suffering from anxiety or deep depression that will definitely affect the family. So, the family is all in this together and need to be open enough to try to understand what this midlife phase means to the women of their household and to their whole family.

The majority of the time husbands will be on the front line of this event. It is a difficult experience for the women and it will also be difficult for their mates. There will be days of tension, moodiness, sadness, crying, and confusion and simply abnormal behavior. There has to be a level of understanding and patience from the husband. They have to go through this together. When she is having anxiety attacks he will probably be participating in calming her or being supportive as he listens to her complain

86

continually about how miserable she is. In most cases men are good sports and need to receive a medal of honor for suffering through this extreme, perplexing time.

Some will even have battle scars. Here are a few examples of encounters one husband may experience any given day or night, i.e.; the woman is having night sweats; she opens the window in the middle of the night then closes it 5 minutes later, or turns the fan on and leaves it on all night so she can sleep, or getting the covers thrown off of him while they are sleeping and its cold. He may also suffer being disturbed often because she is waking up out of her sleep to change wet sleeping garments or just from having a restless night or not being able to touch her body like he used to because the inferno is working overtime and she can't be touched. The woman no longer has interest or desire to be intimate because her libido is very low. While being told that the intimacy that once was great is now the worst that it has ever been because of the pain and discomfort it causes, husbands must sometimes wonder, *Who is this person?* It is not the person they married or fell in love with.

Consequently, there can be a huge strain on the relationship if the connection was not a strong connection prior to the menopausal stages. Men, because there is very little intimacy, will have to go into survival mode. They should understand that it is not about them. She is going through a midlife change and that is the reason for this unusual behavior. But knowing that does not make it any easier.

Couples must discuss what is going on so they can keep the lines of communication open. There are also other loved ones who will encounter this woman who is more difficult or complicated and maybe hard to deal with at times. She may like you one day and dislike you the next. She may make sense to you one day, but be irrational the next. It may seem as if you are dealing with a split personality or two different people.

Most children of a menopausal woman are 9 times out of 10 either teenagers who are very busy and self absorbed or adults who are probably living in their own place and will not have daily contact with their mother. This means most of them don't see what the mother is experiencing. Unless your grandchildren are living with you, they will not witness many of your menopausal episodes. Grandchildren and grandparents have a special bond so there will be very few negative or challenging moments when together. Even if you are experiencing symptoms, when with your grandchildren you will put your best foot forward to enjoy them.

Her Story 10 - Beverly

I remember being in the unemployment office at age 42. I got extremely hot, from head to toe and I looked around to see if anyone else appeared uncomfortable. I asked one of the caseworkers if the air conditioning was on. He responded, "Yes, it is", as he looked at me as if I were a crazy woman. I still have hot flashes today over 20 years later. They were so severe I had to use Premarin and was on it for 2 years when my gynecologist told me she had to take me off of them. So she prescribed a generic brand which did not help at all.

When I went back she increased the dosage and I slept like a baby that night. Then 2 months later I was right back where I started. Sometimes my episodes are so intense they unnerve me.

Even though I had been anticipating hot flashes, when they finally came I was hot and feverish so I thought I was coming down with a virus. I remember what my mother use to say about menopause, "Your body will make a complete change and things will happen to you and you won't know why". Here's a really good example, one day I was driving in my car and I felt like I needed to scream, so I did.

I have some idea what triggers my hot flashes and night sweats so I don't eat as much spicy foods as I used to plus I have changed my overall diet.

Even today, I sleep with the ceiling fan and stand up fan and the air conditioning on simultaneously to stay comfortable. My husband used to complain because it would be too cold in our bed room, now he has adjusted.

During the early stages I had a real attitude problem. I would have extreme mood swings, so to make myself feel better I would shop. I bought a lot of dresses and shoes during that time. If I was having difficulty dealing with coworkers or clients I would leave work early and go shopping. That would allow me to feel good for 3-4 days. I don't have to do that anymore.

I remember when I was at a customer's home and began to have hot flashes. I was sweating so profusely that she had to get me a towel and I had to sit on the floor because I was so hot. I stayed on the floor until I recovered.

Going through menopause affected me emotionally. There were some issues that I was not dealing with, concerns of getting old, unnerving hot flashes, sadness, loneliness and mood-swings, all prompted me to see a counselor. She believed I was over stretched and that I needed to say no. But, I had to raise my children alone while my husband was on the road so that wasn't possible.

Later, we uprooted and moved back home even though I did not want to. That was a real adjustment. Soon after we settled in I had several emergency surgeries. In a very short period of time, I had my gallbladder removed. My intestines wrapped around themselves, so that had to be corrected. Internal scar tissue prevented me from eating and more. It seemed like they just kept finding something seriously wrong. I started to believe that all those years that I did not take care of my body were finally catching up with me. I was now concerned about my mortality. It became obvious that time was winding down for me. I saw 60 as my life expectancy. Now that I am over the 60 mark, I am fighting to stay healthy by making healthy choices.

My mother didn't really talk about menopause with me, because she didn't have any visible symptoms. I never saw her experience hot flashes and she believed mine were so intense because I was so dramatic and made a big deal out of everything.

CHAPTER 10

SHHH... IT'S TABOO

"We're living in an age when people need to talk. They don't communicate"-Queen Latifah

It is common knowledge that years ago when women tried to explain to their physicians what they were going through they were dismissed and told that these feelings were non-existent, all in their heads, or not real. If doctors did take them seriously, they risk the chance of being committed. So, consequently, a generation of women decided not to risk being considered, crazy and just stopped talking about it altogether.

Even today, menopause is generally associated with negative connotations in western cultures. While numerous physical and emotional symptoms have been attributed to it, hot flushes and night sweats are the main physical change. Recent studies suggest that cognitive factors, particularly beliefs about other people's reactions to their hot flashes and night sweats might increase distress, causing embarrassment and behavioral avoidance. Younger men and women tend to have more negative attitudes to menopause.

Menopause has always been a taboo subject. In the past, society has labeled women over 50 as less: less attractive, less important, less valuable or less sexy and this has made self disclosure risky. Women have always wanted to know and understand what these changes mean but they are afraid to ask anyone, it is almost like revealing ones age. She believes once people know her real age they may see her differently. To add insult to injury, society's stigma is, if a woman is going through menopause she is old, past her prime, over the hill, ready to be put out to pasture and many more negativities. Women choose not to announce when they are experiencing any type of symptoms for fear of what people may think. No one wants to be treated as if they are not attractive or more than that, that they no longer matter.

Today, Baby Boomers are a little more open with their discussion on menopause. With help from the media some companies are catching on and have begun to market products that provide relief. With 40 million baby boomers passing through menopause during the next two decades, the taboos are rapidly disappearing.[64]

Yes, it is true, you are no longer of child-bearing age, and no it does not mean that you are useless, insignificant, or over the hill, but it does mean that you are going through the "change", but there is nothing wrong with you. Most Baby Boomers are not willing or ready to wear those labels created by society once worn by women from the 1940's, 50's or even 60's - not willing for fear that they may be viewed as old, elderly or worse, a senior citizen. The reality is they are healthy, vibrant, business women, mothers, grandmothers, teachers, volunteers, creators, travelers, and much more. They want to be respected and viewed for who they are and what they have to offer versus how old they are.

Prime example - Women over 50 are serving in Congress, running for President of the U.S., college presidents, Supreme Court judges, movie producers and directors, and holding high offices. They are also international designers, millionaires, anchor women for major TV networks, successful talk show hosts, and much more and they show no signs of slowing down.

"As a white candle in a holy place, so is the beauty of an aged face." Joseph Campbell

It is universal knowledge that when women age they are called old, but men when they age are called distinguished. That's a double standard.

Media dictated by society affects our conversation they play a big role in menopause continuing to be taboo. We follow the lead of the media, but when we receive the message sent from the media that is where we spend our dollars. Furthermore, if media shows something in a negative light or do not show it at all (omission) we believe them and we see that subject as negative. I realize that was a contradictory statement. But as consumers our dollars influence what media supports but on the other hand, if they provide positive feedback about a subject we believe it is okay and follow their lead.

Face it, women dealing with menopause is not a popular subject. If society glamorized menopause and showed women over 50 confident, vivacious, vibrant, it is my belief that the general populations would change their view of our generation also. They would begin to see them as an extremely important part of society.

Getting back to family communication, information is not passed down within family circles because mothers do not talk about it, grandmothers don't talk about it, the older women in the community, just do not talk about it.

I am sure while growing up I never heard any adults talk about the change and even though I lived at home until age 18. I never ever heard my mother or grandmother mention it and because we respected our adults we did not dare ask them about it. Some days it was obvious there was some discomfort, or anxiety, or unhappiness going on, but no one addressed it. Conversation should begin by age 30. Why wait, reality is that women in their 30's are losing Estrogen and women in their 40's have already begun experiencing one or more symptoms but don't know what it is. If you are not comfortable talking with your young women when they reach puberty than begin during their child bearing years. Teach them early about what is happening with their body and they will understand and be able to deal with it better. Definitely talk before the mental and emotional symptoms such as depression, anxiety and feelings of going crazy have an affect on them.

When discussing it, openly use the words perimenopause, menopause or post menopausal. Conversation could go something like this, *"Jennifer when you see me sweating and uncomfortable I am experiencing what is called hot flashes. Have you heard of them? Well, hot flashes are when my brain tells my body erroneously, that it is cool and it needs warming up and my body tries to accommodate, therefore causing the body to warm up quickly resulting in flashing. This is all as a result of me experiencing menopause. There are many other symptoms associated with menopause, but I wanted to share this with you. If you have any questions about it please come and ask me."* Simple and short explanations like this one will open the door for future conversation.

Who should discuss it? Everyone should discuss it. But, discussion should be led by those who are on the journey, currently in one of the stages of menopause or who have studied about women in the journey such as the medical community, educators, health and wellness facilitators, physicians or other knowledgeable professionals.

Open communications would set women free. If the stigma is removed, the negative connotations would be dropped and everyone could openly discuss it. We would see a different view of the word "menopause".

There needs to be more encouraging images, in commercials, story lines, advertisements, other marketing scenes that deal with midlife issues. Every generation needs to be educated and have an understanding of its purpose. Talking about it openly and respectfully removes the shame and ultimately changes people's attitudes about women over 50.

Media addresses menopause as a medicinal issue versus a relationship, hormonal, physical and mental change or even as a social issue. They could show women with gray hair enjoying life, dating, partying, and traveling, dancing really loving life. Show real women who are 50-60 but still look 40, which is more realistic, who are beautiful, lively and still up on their game with no gray hair.

There is a bright side of maturing. Midlife women experience self confidence, financial stability, happiness, loving family and enjoying grandchildren and being finished with raising children. There is so much to cherish and enjoy at this stage of their lives. That part of a woman's life needs to be conveyed. Furthermore, statistics indicate that women in this time of their lives are happier. Most of the women I interviewed admitted this is a great time for them and they know and like themselves better than when they were younger.

Reading a USA today article written about baby boomers, several things were revealed. I was enlightened by this news. Society needs to take heed;" As Baby Boomers are aging and accumulating wealth, their spending is growing at a pace that's leaving younger generations far behind. Spending by the 116 million U.S. consumers age 50 and older was $2.9 trillion last year — up 45% in the past 10 years. Meanwhile, the 182 million people younger than 50 spent $3.3 trillion last year — up just 6% during the same decade, according to an analysis for USA TODAY the Boomer Project. [65]

And unlike the People 50 and older will inherit an estimated $14 trillion to $20 trillion during the next 20 years." This is something that will never happen again," says Brent Bouchez, founder of consulting firm Agency Five-0, which specializes in adults 50 and older. "What's more, this group will probably not leave a lot of that money to the next generation."… stereotype of older consumers being averse to new things, Boomers are among the biggest buyers of new technology and new cars.[66]

"It s been said that no one can really motivate anyone else; all you can do is instill a positive attitude and hope it catches on"-Eddie Robinson

"It takes only one person to change your life----you." Ruth Casey

Her Story 11 – Karen

At age 42, I experienced erratic menstrual periods. I would go a couple months without a period and when I would have one it would be extremely heavy with severe cramps. I really cried a lot, was happy one minute and 10 minutes later unhappy.

I did things that were uncharacteristic to my personality. I remember one day when I just threw the newspapers on the floor. Another time I kicked a chair. I felt everyone was out to get me. And they had the problem, not me. When my husband put his head in his hands and said he just didn't know what to do to help me and I really felt sorry for him. Then instantly I wanted to slap him for putting his head in his hands. Today I am ashamed to admit how mean I was. My mean behavior lasted for 2-3 years. During that time I was extremely frustrated, hated myself and everyone around me. Nothing made me happy at least not for very long. Other people noticed the change in me and they couldn't understand me, and that would make me angry. But today my symptoms are not that pronounced. I may get warmer than normal on some days or my taste buds seem hard to satisfy sometimes.

My night sweats caused sleepless nights, which added to my aggravation. My son would call me Kathy Bates from the movie Misery. Or ask which witch is Mom today. Good witch or bad witch. I was verbally abusive to my family and friends. My friend who is younger had asked my children what was wrong with their mother.

I did not like my house, it was ugly. I did not participate in things like I used to such as; antiquing, festivals, family gatherings, etc. I lacked motivation. If I went out with the family, I felt I was forced to go.

While I was going through this I went to a family doctor who did various test and ruled out menopause. So I did not know what was wrong with me.

My Mother never did talk to me about menstrual periods or menopause. But I do remember her getting up in the middle of the night and going outside during the winter months because she was experiencing night sweats. I believe if she had of talked to me I would not have been so caught off guard. After 3 years of *experiencing the erratic behavior little by little I began to become myself again. I believe it took a total of 5 years before I went through perimenopause then menopause when my cycle completely stopped. My husband stuck by me through all of this, even though he had never experienced it before.*

Once I figured out what was wrong with me I was pretty much through the journey. I did try taking HT for 3 weeks. Until one day I wasn't feeling well so I went to my Doctor who did blood work and explained that the HT caused the enzymes in my liver to elevate. So I stopped taking them immediately and decided to work through it without help. I believed the worst was over.

Another day I was cutting grass and I started experiencing horrible cramps and some bleeding. I went to the emergency room and the doctor said my uterus was hard so the first thing I thought was, cancer. I went to my gynecologist and he said no the uterus is not hard it is not cancer, it's just menopause. So I was really relieved.

Even though I stopped my cycle by age 47 about 7-8yrs later I had a menstrual break through. One day I was moving bricks that were heavy all by myself and later I noticed spotting and it went into a full cycle. Because I was alarmed I went to my Gynecologist and he did numerous test, paps, etc. and determined there was nothing wrong, however the extreme labor may have brought my period back on temporarily.

CHAPTER 11

WEIGHT LOSS TIPS

Weight gain is a major issue for women from the beginning of their puberty years. The average woman gains 10 pounds per year from the beginning of child bearing through middle age.

If you are serious about losing weight you must commit to a lifestyle change, which includes changing the way you think about food, about exercising and about yourself. You must commit to grocery shopping differently, cooking wiser and eating healthier. It is a lifetime commitment. I have had the opportunity to provide weight loss coaching for women since 2004 and all of the successful clients have embraced the philosophy of making a complete lifestyle change.

How to lose weight

First of all, I would like to emphasize that I do not believe in going on diets. It is my opinion that they are designed for short term results and for most women dieting is a sure way to fail. There are two main elements to losing weight and that is your diet (eating plan) and exercise regimen. I always share the (PZ Elite) eating plan when I do presentations because it was designed by someone very dear to me and more than that I know it works. And lastly, as a result of one of the meals, individuals who follow this plan find relief from some of their menopause symptoms.

This plan includes the following; carbohydrates and soy protein drink to start your day, chicken and fish with fruits and vegetable and of course grains. It's a well rounded meal approach that teaches discipline and healthy eating. The plan is designed to jump start your metabolism so you should not be on it long term. But the three weeks you are on it there should be some weight loss.

Follow an existing, proven plan, don't be creative and do your own thing. My hypothesis is that if what you were doing in the past worked; you wouldn't need to have a weight loss plan in the first place. Currently, there's a large number of weight loss programs, healthy eating plans, diets, slim down plans, and so on out there already. Find a healthy, credible plan that works for you and fits within your lifestyle. If you enjoy the plan and it fits you are more likely to stick with it long term.

You have to include exercising in this plan to burn those unwanted calories or units of energy. Which ultimately if not burned turns to fat and is stored in your body.

Every individual is at a different level when it comes to the need for exercising. First, look at stretching. It has been suggested for individuals over a certain age and sedentary (couch potato), but if that does not apply to you then you do not have to read on. For the majority of you getting up in the morning and starting the day stretching provides flexibility of bones, joints, muscles etc. If you are beyond stretching develop a more intense plan.

When to exercise-Day or night is okay. If you exercise mornings it gives you energy to make it through the day if you exercise in the evening it may help you sleep better at night.

I use to exercise during my lunch hour because it was a de-stressor for me and by doing that I handled stressful situations and circumstances healthier. I would always appear cool, calm and collective because I worked out my stress and left it in the gym. More companies are offering Wellness programs in addition to offering incentives to exercise while at work. There are stats that an employee who practices healthy habits is a healthier employee and saves the company money.

Follow these 9 easy steps:

1. Do some research and select an eating plan. Don't choose just any plan make sure it is something that works for you. FOR EXAMPLE-Bob Greene (Oprah's Coach), Pz Elite, Dr. Ian (Million pound weight loss challenge) There are hundreds of plans out there, just select the one you believe in. Look for a plan that includes; lean meats, fruits and vegetables, grains and healthy carbohydrates.

2. Secondly, remove all those foods from your kitchen that are not going to benefit you. Empty the pantry, the refrigerator, and anywhere else you hide food. You are weak and easy to falter and you do not want to be tempted. Give them away or throw them away, just do not keep them in the house.

3. Next create a list before going to the store which include only those food items in your plan, then shop for those healthy foods that are listed in your plan. If it is not on your list do not purchase it. This includes reading labels.

4. Planning and meal preparation is key. Prepare several meals in advance, package them, and heat up when it is time to eat. Preparation is the key to success. If you had a long day at work or with the kids, you come home hungry and tired and all you have to do is take your meal out of the refrigerator or freezer, heat and eat then you will be more likely to eat a healthy meal.

5. Remember If It Is Not on the Plan...Do No Eat It.
6. Map out your exercise plan-workout 4-5 days every week, no excuses.
7. Drink lots of water. There are two schools of thought that you should drink 6 -8 oz of water daily or calculate it according to your body weight to determine how much you should drink. Either way it is vital to hydrate your body with water.
8. Eat your last meal before 7 p.m., 8p.m at latest. You need to give your body an opportunity to begin the digestion process before going to bed. That is why you have heard it is not healthy to eat and go right to bed.
9. Eat 4-5 times per day. This is a time when more is better. It is a myth to eat less or starve yourself to lose weight. You must feed your body so it will have calories to burn off.

Other valuable health and wellness tips:

1.   There are several things that go along with being overweight this time of your life. You need to be concerned with what is going on inside your body. Statistically if you are overweight there's a greater chance that you will have one or more of the following illnesses in your lifetime: high cholesterol; high blood pressure; heart disease; and/or diabetes
2.   Be smart Know your numbers - According to Health and Human Services; to be determined healthy your numbers should be within the following range:
BMI -18-25 is on target, 25.5-29 is classified as overweight, over 30 is obese with glucose below 100 and blood pressure-120/85

Cholesterol - There are two types of cholesterol: "good" and "bad". It is important to understand the difference and to know the levels of good and bad cholesterol in your blood. Too much of one type or not enough of another can put one at risk for coronary heart disease, heart attack or stroke. If your total cholesterol score is less than 200 mg/dL and you have none of the above-mentioned risk factors, you are at low risk for heart disease. A total cholesterol score of 200-239 mg/DL is considered borderline high and anything above that is considered high. [67]
The lower your LDL (bad) cholesterol, the lower your risk of heart attack and stroke.

"I don't believe in failure. It is not failure if you enjoyed the process"- Oprah Winfrey

"So many people are afraid of taking even the smallest chance. They cling to dull routines as if those routines are life rafts."- Overheard at Juniors restaurant in Brooklyn

Time to Make that Lifestyle change - How to make the lifestyle change- Losing weight is not only about dropping pounds but also changing the way you think about what you do and how you do it. It is about making a commitment to doing things differently. First of all change is defined as; verb to become different, or make something or somebody different; transitive verb to exchange, substitute, or replace something (Encarta Dictionary) online.

Change is extremely difficult for most people. They are satisfied as long as they are allowed to continue doing things the way they have always done it, even though the results or consequences may be disastrous.

When I talk about making a lifestyle change I emphasize that it is a long term journey and you will be on this journey for the rest of your life. It is what it says "lifestyle change" you are a participant throughout your lifetime. When people determine they are ready to change they must first get their minds in order. After the mind has made the commitment, the rest will follow. This is a vital step because until you receive that revelation your weight will go up and down, and never meet your goals. Anything that encompasses food you will now do differently. Once you are able to do that you will continue to lose weight and not gain it back. And when you reach your goal you will be able to maintain your weight.

"The measure of success is not whether you have a tough problem to deal with but whether it is the same problem you had last year."
- John Foster Dulles

Her Story 12 – Lucy

I was always the type of person to practice preventative medicine. I began to have an extremely heavy menstrual period around age 50. I went to my OBGYN to find out why this was happening and what to do about it. I was having periods 7-14 days nonstop then it increased even more and the doctor said I was losing too much blood and that I should consider a hysterectomy. This went on for two years before I agreed to have the surgery and immediately he put me on a hormone replacement therapy called Premarin. He looked very closely at my family history and saw there was no cancer there so he put me on a low dosage.

Since I went on Premarin right away I never experienced any menopausal symptoms and because it was believed that Premarin could cause cancer, my doctor monitored me closely. I would get blood work done every three months, regular pap smears and breast exams and I still do that even today. During that time I would see a heart specialist every year because there was some concern about women over 50 getting heart disease. I still do this today.

I took Premarin for about 13 years until age 65. When I went off of the medication I had no symptoms to contend with. But my mother never had hot flashes or any visible menopausal symptoms, and one of my sisters who has never had a hysterectomy or ever experienced menopausal symptoms to speak of either. Of course, it doesn't mean there are not other things going on inside our bodies that we can't see.

I always lived a perfect, stress- free life. I had a super husband and a great child. I came from a close knit family with a father who was a great provider, a mother who was a great teacher and my life has always been wonderful.

As an adult I always had great opportunities. I was in high school during WWII when given the opportunity to go to Anderson College to train for a government job. You see, all the men were fighting in the war. After college they offered me a job in Dayton at WPAFB. I was assigned to commissioned military personnel from 1944-1960. Then late in life I went home to have and raise my first child.

After three years, I was recruited to work for a major GM company as the Affirmative Action Coordinator. My job was to track the number of minorities (Blacks and Women) in the city available to work. At that time out of 14,000 employees there was only one Black supervisor and 3% women in the company and before I retired I had become supervisor of Personnel services.

I left GM but not the workforce at age 61 I went to work for the Ohio Civil rights commission and stayed there for 10 years and retired a second time.

I was always deeply rooted in the community, from having my own show on a new local radio station to volunteering on numerous committees and organizations. I wanted to help those families in need. Many times my contribution entailed raising money to operate programming to better our community.

I served with organizations such as: American Cancer Society, YMCA, United Negro College Fund, County Children Services Board, NAACP, and many more. It constantly kept me very busy but I did it because I always enjoyed serving people.

CHAPTER 12

GOOD OLE GIRLS SUPPORT GROUP

Koch and Mansfield (2004) noted that women need to avoid overextending themselves in providing support to others and need to focus instead on getting the support they need. Koch and Mansfield emphasized three forms of social support: informational support (information and advice), emotional support (empathy and caring), and instrumental support (tangible aid and services).

Although counselors and other health care professionals are clear sources of support, a major form of self-care involves reaching out to current support networks of family and friends and, perhaps, extending social networks through support groups and online resources.[67]

The many changes that occur during menopause, combined with the confusion and fear associated with it will make this a troubling time for some women. We believe counselors are in a unique position to provide accurate biomedical information within an integrative approach that conceptualizes menopause as a normative midlife transition.[68]

I'm sure you are aware of the saying: "Good ole Boys club", well it is time to have an all girls Menopause club. I am advocating that women all over the nation come together and begin sharing in small groups their experiences. Talking about thoughts, feelings, anecdotes, commonalities, likes, dislikes and so on. Support groups have been around for hundreds of years and are extremely important, case in point, there's; Alcoholics Anonymous, Jenny Craig, Weight Watchers, and all of these groups were created because someone had a need and found others who had a common issue and determined if they work through those items together in groups more people are helped. Creating universality is so important.

How to begin your group per Corey and Corey – There are practical considerations in forming a group. Below are a few examples:

Group composition - In general, for a specific target population with given needs, a group composed entirely of members of that population is more appropriate than a heterogeneous group. This similarity of the members can lead to a great degree of cohesion, which in turn allows for an open and intense exploration of their life crises. Members can express feelings that they typically withhold and their life circumstances can give then a bond with one another.

Group size - It depends on several factors; for a weekly ongoing group of adults, about 8 people may be ideal. A group of this size is big enough to give ample opportunity for interaction and small enough for everyone to be involved and to feel a sense of "group". Corey and Corey also addresses whether it should be an open versus closed group. Open groups are characterized by changing membership. As certain members leave, new members are admitted and the group continues. Closed typically have some time limitation with the group meeting for a predetermined number of sessions. Generally, members are expected to remain in the group until it ends and new members are not added. [70]

How do you benefit? - It is always beneficial to have a place you can go and discuss personal issues that you are very concerned about and not have to worry about confidentiality. Not only are you able to discuss openly in group, but you will hear from others what they are going through and how they've handled their menopausal experiences past or present. You'll experience commonality- which means that others are going through the same issues you are. You begin to realize that you are not strange or weird, because others have some of the same issues and in addition to that you get tips on what to do about it. For example one member may share that she has always had a cup of coffee before going to bed because it calms her and allows her to wind down but can't understand why she is having night sweats to the point where she has to change her clothes at night. Someone may suggest to her from experience that that caffeine is a sure trigger for hot flashes and can lead to intense night sweats. As the participants share how they are handling their experiences, it is very settling to find camaraderie in your experiences.

Recruiting - Talk to women who may be experiencing menopause or who know someone who is. Get volunteers.

Why it is necessary? - Too much is at stake this is imperative. By nature women congregate in groups, they talk with a circle of friends when they need advice, they join clubs or organizations, they hang out in pairs, they are more like packs. So participating in a support group is not unusual for them. Once again it provides support and commonality.

"Excessive or prolonged stress, particularly in the form of frustration, fear or anxiety is distress and leads to disease". Hail C. Christopher

CHAPTER 13

TIPS FOR QUICK RELIEF...
and Old-Time Remedies To Assist You Through The Process

I have provided a few quick menopausal relief recommendations including my famous menopause survival kit. These tips derived from talking to several women about what works for them in addition to my own personal techniques. There is nothing scientific about them, but they are working for some:

The *Yes, Real Women Do Sweat* survival kit - Keep this with you at all times:

- Tweezers -to pluck unwanted hairs
- Extra pair of panties for continence(leakage)
- A fan paper or battery operated. Something small enough to carry in your purse-for those hot flashes
- Bottled water- to stay cool
- A sweater or small wrap
- Pictures of family and friends, so you do not forget them

On the serious side these tips are extremely helpful:

a) Be conscious of your clothing -If you dress too warm by wearing too many layers or if your fabric holds in body heat you could trigger hot flashes. Dress lightly in cottons (because they breathe) with short sleeves when appropriate, and carry a sweater or jacket for when you feel a chill.

b) Don't sleep in a hot room -keep your environment at a comfortable temperature, moderate heat or air conditioning to keep at a cool temperature. This decreases night sweats and insomnia. For example, at night during the winter months, before retiring turn heat down to 64-65degrees. "Smile" I know that is a joke for some of you, but this suggestion actually came from my family doctor in the early 1990's.

c) When you feel you are having an anxiety attack or your heart is palpitating fast, stop what you are doing and take several deep breaths, count to 10, sit and relax for a minute and take a sip of cold water. If it continues see a doctor.

d) Exercise to keep the body flexible and strong. Helps to keep stress and anxiety down. Walk, run, do aerobics, whatever you choose, just move that body. If you are at work stop and take a short break and walk. Remember exercises releases endorphins which cause you to feel good.

e) Mentally exercise and challenge your brain daily to increase alertness and decrease fogginess and forgetfulness. Play crossword puzzles, word games, math games, read etc.

f) Become more aware of personal wants and needs and take better care of yourself you deserve it.

g) If you are a smoker know that statistics show women who smoke have more intense hot flashes than women who do not. Plus it causes cancer and increases the risk of heart disease. So stop smoking.

h) When you are suffering from a hot flashes just use cold water. Go to a faucet and run cold water on your hands, put some on your neck and face if possible, also drink a tall glass of ice cold water until you feel relief.

i) Talk about it-Open up to friends, strangers, family whoever will listen. Sometimes there is liberation from self disclosure about what you are experiencing.

j) Laugh-Laughter does the body and mind good- "One of the problems with reconnecting with your sense of humor and your sense of fun is that you have to remember what kinds of things use to make you laugh out loud. They don't even have to be funny; there're just odd, unexpected, unusual, and frequently stupid. It would probably help you make a list of all kinds of things that you can count on to make you laugh and post it somewhere you'll see it every day. [70]

A familiar quote from Maya Angelou " *When you know better you do better*".

CHAPTER 14

RESOURCES
Medical Findings, Resources and Updates

Often, I talked about the importance of being intelligent about what is going on in your life and the best way to do that is through research. The first place to find great information on every topic is on the internet by searching the worldwide web.

Use Goggle advance search, Bing, or Yahoo or the most current search engine. Then specify what you are looking for by using words and phrases and you can dig into a world of information from the matches you will receive.

The second and definitely not least is your public library. There is still a tremendous amount of information written by the Medical community, research organizations such as the National Institute of Health Initiative. The library has a research and data section on line that allows you to pull up the most recent findings and articles written on any topic.

Also, interview women who are experiencing menopause themselves so you get a personal perspective. Dialoguing is crucial, each person has her own experiences and a wealth of information and would probably be grateful that you were interested enough to elicit conversation. Sometimes we can learn more from each other.

If you are interested in focusing more on the medical aspect then use your local University libraries in addition to the public library. Many books, research papers, presentation papers, Clinical studies, case studies, articles have been written about the effects of menopause, but it is up to you to seek out to find the information. If you do not have a local University, search the libraries online. Using an extensive search you can find everything you need to know about menopause.

Before you begin your search, be clear on what you are trying to find out. Once you determine that, use headings or phrases like; symptoms of menopause or explaining menopause, Medical updates on menopause, local resources for menopausal women, effects of menopause, living with menopause, hot flashes and menopause, etc. If that is too broad, narrow the search down and be more specific.

If you use the Advance search by Google you can use words that will narrow it down to exactly what you are looking for.

Don't be ignorant about this topic. To be empowered you need knowledge because it is true that "Knowledge is Power". Keep current on findings and updates. We are always hoping for good answers that will help women live a better quality of life and will provide more explanations on why our body behaves the way it does, and what we can do to combat some of those negative symptoms. As more money is poured into research, ideals change. What was true a decade ago may no longer be true. What we thought was true a century ago has been proven incorrect this century. The more you know the better your life will be.

Menopause Resources

Office on Women's Health, HHS
200 Independence Ave. SW, Room 712E
Washington, D.C. 20201
http://www.womenshealth.gov/owh

National Heart, Lung, and Blood Institute, NIH, HHS
P.O Box 30105
Bethesda, MD 20824
http://www.nhlbi.nih.gov

Office of Research on Women's Health, CDC, HHS
1600 Clifton Rd, NE, MS E-89
Atlanta, GA 30333
http://www.cdc.gov/women/

Oesteoporosis and Related Bone Disease National Resource
Center, NIH, HHS
2 AMS Circle
Bethesda, MD 20892
http://www.niams.nih.gov/Health_Info/Bone/

American Menopause Foundation, Inc.
350 5th Avenue, Suite 2822
New York, NY 10118
http://www.americanmenopause.org

Black Women's Health Imperative
1420 K Streey, N.W. Suite 1000
Washington, DC 20036
http://**www.blackwomenshealth.org**

National Women's Health Network
514 10th Strery, NW, Suite 400

Washington, DC 20004
http://www.nwhn.org

North American Menopause Society (NAMS)
P.O. Box 94527
Cleveland, OH 44101
http://www.menopause.org/

Quiz

Take this short fun quiz to see if you pass. ...Read each scenario and choose the answer that best describes what you would do. Even though these scenarios were created just for this book some of them may sound familiar to you. What would you do? There really is no right answer. I am trying to teach you how to be more accepting of menopause, more confident, self-assured and confident in your state of mind.

1.   You are in a meeting and you sense a hot flash coming on, do you?

   a) Ignore it and hope it goes away
   b) Begin fanning to cool off quickly
   c) Leave the room before it comes on
   d) Drink your cold pop(soda) to cool off

2.   You dropped your ink pen but each time you reach for it, it rolls out of your reach, do you?

   a) Leave it on the floor
   b) Ask someone else to pick it up
   c) Focus totally on picking up the ink pen
   d) Kick the ink pen

3.   You are in the middle of a conversation at a networking session and you begin to have an anxiety attack do you?

   a) Keep talking through the anxiety episode
   b) Stop talking to allow calming yourself down
   c) Walk away in the middle of the conversation
   d) Tell them what is going on

4. While visiting a friend you are offered one of your favorite beverages, but from experience you know you will have intense hot flashes, do you?

a) Refuse the beverage and explain why
b) Request water or another safe drink
c) Do you accept the drink because its your favorite
d) Accept it so you won't appear rude

5. You are out with friends and no one at your table appears to be warm but you, do you?

a) Ask whether anyone else is warm
b) Assume no one else is hot and make moves towards cooling your body off
c) Ignore it to keep from bringing attention to yourself
d) Ask the owner of the establishment if the air conditioning is working

6. You are in a car with coworkers and you sense a hot flash coming on, (in the dead of winter), do you?

a) Ask permission to let the window down
b) Begin fanning to cool off
c) Bring attention to yourself by joking about what you are going through
d) All the above

7. You can not remember the last name of an old friend, but you want to introduce them to a new friend, do you?

a) Do not introduce them at all
b) Introduce them using first names only
c) Ask for forgiveness and ask the old friend to give her last name
d) Don't sweat it (this time) everyone forgets names

8.   You are in the middle of a presentation and your entire thought escapes you, do you?

   a) Skip it and go back to it
   b) Verbally acknowledge that you lost your thought and pick it up at the next point
   c) Try to recall the information even though it may take you a while
   d) Pretend like nothing happened

9. You are working intensely on a project when you begin to feel anxious and claustrophobic, do you?

   a) Stop what you are doing a hot flash is probably on the way
   b) Work through it those feelings will eventually go away
   c) Tell someone because maybe you are having a breakdown
   d) Turn on some music

10. You are losing your patience because you had to repeat your instructions to a family member several times and they still can't seem to get it right, do you?

   a) Blow your top maybe this time they will get it
   b) Walk away from the person something is obviously wrong with them
   c) Write down the instructions and let them read them
   d) Calm down, collect your thoughts and very calmly explain the instructions in elementary terms, even show them how it's done if necessary

These are my answers: 1(b) 2(b or c) 3(b) 4(a and b) 5(b) 6(d) 7(b and d) 8(b) 9(a) 10(d)

REFERENCES/BIBLIOGRAPHY

http://www.metlife.com/assets/cao/mmi/publications/st udies/mmi-studies-boomer-profile-2007.pdf, A Profile of American Baby Boomers was prepared by MetLife's Mature Market InstituteSM.

http://www.livestrong.com/article/8774-need-length-menopause/#ixzz1SCL4I9ll

Menopause for Dummies, by Marcia L. Jones, PhD, Theresa Eichenwald, MD, and Nancy W. Hall, Wiley Publishing, Inc. 2007

http://www.umm.edu/altmed/articles/spirituality-000360.htm

Menopause for Dummies by Marcia L. Jones, PhD, Theresa Eichenwald, MD, and Nancy W. Hall, Wiley Publishing, Inc. 2007

http://www.sciencedirect.com/science/article/pii/S009082 5800960104

http://womenshealth.gov/menopause/early-premature-menopause/

http://nmhn.org/hysterectomy2005

Menopause for dummies by Marcia L. Jones, PhD, Theresa Eichenwald, MD, and Nancy W. Hall, Wiley Publishing, Inc. 2007

Women Bodies, Women Wisdom; Creating Physical & Emotional Health & Healing by Dr.Christiane

Northrup, Bantam Books, NY, Copyright 1994 revised 2010

http://www.livestrong.com/article/8774-need-length-menopause/#ixzz1SCNTMsRw

http://www.power-surge.com/headlines/hotflash.htm

http://www.breastcancer.org/tips/menopausal/facing/hot_flashes.jsp

http://www.segweb.org/index.php/langen/component/content/article/101-atrophie-urogenitale?

Urogenital atrophy J. Calleja-Agius and M. P. Brincat
    Women Bodies, Women Wisdom; Creating Physical & Emotional Health & Healing by Dr. Christiane Northrup, Bantam Books, NY, Copyright 1994 revised 2010

Menopause: The Journal of the North American Menopause Society. Vol.14no3pp 357-369 2007

Johnston SL, Farrell SA, Bouchard C, et al. The detection and management of vaginal atrophy. J Obstet Gynaecol Can 2004;26:503–15

http://www.minniepauz.com/menopause-symptom-dry-vagina.html

Women Bodies, Women Wisdom; Creating Physical & Emotional Health & Healing by Dr. Christiane Northrup, Bantam Books, NY, Copyright 1994 revised 2010

http://www.epigee.org/menopause/palpitations.html

http://www.doctoroz.com/search?q1=When+was+the+palpitation+due+to+Menopause+on%3F

http://www.mayoclinic.com/health/heartdisease/HB00040

http://www.nhlbi.nih.gov/educational/hearttruth/lower-risk/risk-factors.htm

http://www.nhlbi.nih.gov/actintime/haws/women.htm

http://www.webmd.com/osteoporosis/bone-mineral-density?page=3

Quinn M. Pearson, Department of Counselor Education, University of North Alabama. Correspondence, University of North Alabama, UNA Box 5154, Elorence, AL 35632 (e-mail: qmpearson@una.edu). 76 ADULTSPAN/oarW Ealt2010 Vol.9 No. 2

http://uhs.berkeley.edu/lookforthesigns/depressionsuicide.shtml

http://www.mayoclinic.com/health/low-sex-drive-in-women/DS01043/DSECTION=causes

http://www.mayoclinic.com/health/low-sex-drive-in-women/DS01043

http://www.mayoclinic.com/health/low-sex-drive-in-women/DS01043

http://www.skinlaser.com/skin-conditions-washington-dc/
http://www.webmd.com/healthy-beauty/features/age-dry-skin

http://www.nhlbi.nih.gov/health/dci/Diseases/inso/inso
_whatis.html

Women Bodies, Women Wisdom; Creating Physical &
Emotional Health & Healing by Dr.Christiane
Northrup, Bantam Books, NY, Copyright 1994 r
evised 2010

http://www.mayoclinic.com/health/dry-eyes/DS00463

http://www.menopauserx.com/health_center/sym_facial_
hair.htm

http://www.gallbladderattack.com/sugarcravings.shtml

http://www.nutritionmd.org/consumers/renal/uti.html

http://www.umm.edu/patiented/articles/what_risk_facto
rs_urinary_tract_infections__000036_4.htm

http://www.urbandictionary.com/define.php?term=muffin
%20top

http://www.helpguide.org/life/healthy_diet_fats.htm

Menopause for dummies by Marcia L. Jones, PhD, Theresa
Eichenwald, MD, and Nancy W. Hall, Wiley
Publishing, Inc. 2007
The National Association of Menopause(NAM)-Obstet
Gynecol magazine in 2008

http://www.cancer.gov/cancertopics/understandingcancer
/estrogenreceptors/page3
Counseling Women in Midlife: An Integrative Approach
to Menopause. By: Huffman, Shirley B., Myers, Jane

E., Journal of Counseling & Development, 07489633, Summer99, Vol. 77, Issue 3

Judy R. Strauss CCC Code: 0360-7283/11 ©2011 National Association of Social Workers

Menopause Symptoms and Attitudes of African American Women: Closing the Knowledge Gap and Expanding Opportunities for Counseling Journal article by Shirley B. Huffman, Jane E. Myers, Lynne R. Tingle, Lloyd A. Bond; Journal of Counseling and Development, Vol. 83, 2005

Menopause for dummies by Marcia L. Jones, PhD, Theresa Eichenwald, MD, and Nancy W. Hall, Wiley Publishing, Inc. 2007

"What Color Is Your Diet?: Color Code Foods Made Easy" by Dr. Heber ,Harper with Susan Bowerman,Collins Publishing Co. Regan Books. New York,NY, 2001

http://ods.od.nih.gov/factsheets/vitamind/

http://ods.od.nih.gov/factsheets/VitaminB12-QuickFacts/

http://www.mayoclinic.com/health/fish-oil/NS_patient-fishoil

http://www.healthcastle.com/black-cohosh-menopause.shtml

http://www.healthcastle.com/flax.shtml

http://www.healthline.com/health-slideshow/menopause-perimenopause/depression-and-irritability
http://www.mayoclinic.com/health/dongquai/NS_patient-Dongquai

http://www.insomnia.net/natural-remedies/valarian/

http://www.holisticonline.com/remedies/hrt/hrt_herbs_fo
r_menopause.htm

http://www.picturehistory.com/product/id/18974

http://www.drugs.com/premarin.html

http://www.nlm.nih.gov/medlineplus/ency/article/00711
1.htm

5900 Landerbrook Drive, Suite 390, Mayfield Heights, OH,
44124 / info@menopause.org /440/442-7550

http://www.360menopause.com/blog/tag/hormone-
patches

http://www.menopause.org/hormonetherapystats.aspx

http://www.redhotmamas.org/pdf/good_housekeeping_0
61997.pdf

USA TODAY of U.S. Bureau of Labor Statistics data by The
Boomer Project.

http://www.mediabistro.com/agencyspy/boomers-swarm-
chicago_b5952

http://www.everydayhealth.com/heart-
disease/cholesterol/high-cholesterol-and-heart-
disease.aspx

http://periodicals.faqs.org/201010/2169470381.html

Learning to love menopause. By: Span, Paula, Good
Housekeeping, 0017209X, Jun97, Vol. 224, Issue 6

Corey & Corey Group Therapy book

How'd all These Ping Pong Balls Get in my Bag? By Leigh Ann Jashjeway, MPH and Comedy Workout Publishing

APPENDIX

Breakfast				
Snack				
Lunch				
Snack				
Dinner				
Snack				

REFLECTIONS:

Editor's Note

When Linda Hawkins approached me about editing a book on the topic of menopause, I honestly was not enthused about doing so. I prefer to edit works of fiction and fantasy as I enjoy getting caught up in the world of "make believe". I was sure that editing a book on menopause would become a long and drawn out process and I would need to take many breaks from the material as I was sure it would produce a serious degree of ennui.

From the first page of the book to the last, though, I found myself surprisingly engaged in the content. Matters I was sure would not pertain to me accurately described occurrences in my life. Until I read this book, for which I can completely relate, I thought I might need to see a professional for support. Now, I understand that all of the symptoms I have been experiencing are normal and that many women are going through the same issues.

Linda Hawkins' book, *Yes, Real Women Do Sweat*, is a much needed companion for women who suspect they might be going through menopause or who have had it confirmed they actually are. Like many women, I have been suffering from the symptoms noted in Hawkins' book. Night sweats, memory fogginess, irritability, weight gain, fatigue, nonchalance, and so many more issues have been plaguing my life and until recently, I had no understanding as to why. Not only did Linda's book enlighten me to the indicators of menopause, but also to the preliminary symptoms that affect those of us who are unsuspecting as we are not yet in the prime of the menopausal phase. Hawkins' book is necessary for all women, whether menopause at this time is an issue for them or not. It is also a fantastic and essential guide for men to assist them in understanding the perimenopausal, menopausal, and post menopausal women in their lives. Those terms are clearly defined within the book.

——

Men who are experiencing frustrations with the women in their lives would benefit from gaining an understanding of their women's internal battles. As I edited this book, I shared excerpts of it with my husband, who because of the content has developed a greater understanding and as a result, a greater sensitivity towards me. This book could save your relationship! Don't spend too much time stressing over or researching the issues of menopause. Linda Hawkins has done that for you! *Yes, Real Women Do Sweat,* is one of those books that has earned a right to be on everyone's bookshelves.

With Sincerity,
Dorinda D. E. Nusum
Award-Winning Author of
Afflicted and *The Back Pew Crew*

About The Author

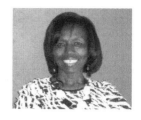

Linda Hawkins is a wife, mother to two adult daughters, and a grandmother of six who loves to teach about Health and Wellness through writing, presentations, and workshops. Linda, one of four children, was born and raised in Michigan. She later married and moved to Dayton, Ohio where she currently resides.

Hawkins received a Bachelors degree in Family Life Specialist at Eastern Michigan University and a Master's degree from Wright State University in Dayton, Ohio. She served eight years as a counselor at a community college where she assisted students in creating their educational plans of action so they might achieve a two-year Health Career Associate's degree. For 10 years, Hawkins served as a Project Director and designed a pre-college program. She went on to become an entrepreneur and opened a local souvenir and old fashioned candy store. A few years later, Hawkins returned to the community college setting as a faculty member.

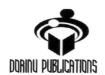

DORINU PUBLICATIONS

Made in the USA
San Bernardino, CA
18 July 2019